AVOID MEDICAL-BILL STICKER SHOCK—FOREVER!

• • •

For years, doctors have urged us to take control of our own health care through preventive measures like exercise, diet, and right living.

Now, it's time we take control of our health care finances—through preventive measures like due diligence and common sense. Assuming responsibility for the accuracy of your medical bill is right living too.

Don't:

- Let health care providers bully you just because you're too sick to fight
- Get bluffed into paying for things you don't owe
- Agree to pay as you go
- Take no for an answer

Do:

- Get an itemized bill for all procedures
- Shop around and compare prices
- Leverage what you know with your hosp
- Take   care

THE MEDICAL BILL

SURVIVAL GUIDE

What You Need to Know Before You Pay a Dime

PAT PALMER
with **MARTHA ELLIS** and
CHRISTOPHER SLONE

WARNER BOOKS

A Time Warner Company

While all the case histories discussed in *The Medical Bill Survival Guide* are true, names and other identifying characteristics have been changed to protect the privacy of the patients and their families.

This book is designed to provide competent and reliable information regarding the subject matter covered. However, it is sold with the understanding that the author and publisher are not engaged in rendering medical or other professional advice. Laws and practices often vary from state to state, and if expert assistance is required, the services of a professional should be sought. The author and publisher specifically disclaim any liability that is incurred from the use or application of the contents of this book.

WARNER BOOKS EDITION

Cover design by Elaine Groh
Book design by Charles S. Sutherland

Warner Books, Inc.
1271 Avenue of the Americas
New York, NY 10020

Visit our Web site at
www.twbookmark.com

 A Time Warner Company

Printed in the United States of America

First Printing: August 2000

10 9 8 7 6 5 4 3 2 1

Acknowledgments

This book is dedicated to all the individuals who had the strength to stand up and fight for their rights. Thanks to Chris Slone for having faith in us and the services we provide for consumers.

Pat Palmer and Martha Ellis

A very special thanks to Dr. Bob Slosser, Dr. John Lawing, Dr. Doug Tarpley, Dr. Terry Lindvall, and Mr. Jeff Deaton, who saw things I didn't.

Chris Slone

Contents

APPENDIX B

Prologue

Mr. Powell's Companion

William Powell didn't need a Ph.D. in mathematics to see that things didn't add up.

Having undergone successful heart surgery a few weeks earlier, the forty-seven-year-old contractor was now staring down at a hospital bill that said he owed $17,248 more than his insurance policy would cover.

No. This can't be right! he thought to himself.

William couldn't believe the amount they were asking for, much less pay it. He had never had anything more serious than the flu before this heart attack struck.

He picked up the phone and dialed the hospital. The billing department there told him that if he thought his bill was wrong, they'd be more than happy to review it for him. He asked them to please do so.

After double-checking the bill, the hospital told William that indeed they had made some mistakes. *Thank God!* he thought to himself, feeling the heavy burden beginning to lift.

But then the hospital went on to tell him he actually owed about $500 *more* than he was originally billed!

William nearly suffered a relapse.

Not knowing what else to do, he did the unthinkable. He decided to question his hospital bill.

William began his investigation by requesting a line-by-line, itemized list of all the specific charges he had incurred during his brief hospital stay. (On closer inspection, the "bill" the hospital originally sent him only told him what to pay, not what it was he was paying *for*.) The hospital seemed a bit annoyed by his request, but they complied.

Immediately William realized he was at another disadvantage. Not only did he lack a doctorate in math, he had never studied medicine, nor had he been trained in decryption by the CIA. The itemized statement he had been given was filled with gibberish like "CKMB" and "ABG + K + " and "ANTI EMBOLI HOSE THIGH M REG."

Worse still, the only item he clearly understood, "MISCELLANEOUS," cost him $27,000!

The miscellaneous charges notwithstanding, it was a less expensive item that actually brought William to my office. Listed on his bill as a "COUGH SUPPORT DEVICE," it had cost him $57.50.

What's a cough support device?

You may not want to know.

Following his surgery, William had awoken in the intensive care unit with a little teddy bear tucked beneath his arm. Like most teddy bears, it was cute, brown, and furry. It had little black eyes and a little black nose. *How sweet,*

William remembered thinking at first. *A get-well present from the staff!*

He was only half right.

The bear *was* from the hospital, but it was no present. "Cough Buddy," William discovered, was the cough support device, a polyester pillow in the form of a bear that the hospital had bought for about $10 and passed along to William for almost $60. (Before hospitals started using and charging for teddy bears like Cough Buddy, patients were able to use ordinary pillows.)

The point is William hadn't asked for the bear. William's doctor had never ordered the bear. William didn't need the bear. But William got the bear.

Boy, did he get it.

And that bear wasn't all that was stuffed into his bill, either.

1

Nine Times out of Ten

WHY THIS BOOK HAD TO BE WRITTEN

More and more people like William Powell are learning that while our health care providers may be treating us well as patients, they're treating us horribly as customers. Reliable studies show that more than *nine out of ten* medical bills contain errors—bills coming from hospitals, from health maintenance organizations (HMOs), from physical therapists, from laboratories, and from everyday visits to the doctor.

Not surprisingly, the error almost always favors those *sending* the bill, not the one receiving it.

One study, done by Equifax Services, puts the average dollar amount of error at around *$1,300 per patient*.

Of course, in times past, the average patient didn't need to concern himself with such misbillings. If an insurance policy said it would cover 80 percent of the total medical costs, it probably did. If and when a health care provider screwed up, the insurance company paid for the mistakes, not the patient. Rarely would an insured patient need to worry about picking up unexpected unpaid tabs.

No longer. With insurance companies and health maintenance organizations privately negotiating fees with hospitals and other medical facilities while at the same time dramatically limiting the amount they will pay for certain procedures, patients are frequently left holding sizable bags themselves.

MY OWN EXPERIENCE

My own experience in investigating medical bills over the last fifteen years only reinforces what the studies are now showing. In fact, I've found the percentage of bills with errors to be higher than 90 percent. Our office alone recovers hundreds of thousands of dollars annually in wrongful billings.

For example, one woman you'll meet shortly saw her out-of-pocket hospital expenses reduced from $20,000 to less than $2,000. Another woman saw the $17,000 cost of her *twenty-three-hour* hospital stay cut in half—within a matter of hours. Other case studies we'll discuss are no less dramatic.

GHOSTS IN THE MACHINE

Name any other type of business that could survive that sort of gross incompetence in the way it bills its customers. I doubt you can. Business executives outside of health care who tolerate such mismanagement not only risk going under.

They risk going to jail.

When I first began finding errors in people's medical bills, I operated under the naive assumption that everyone—hospital administrators, doctors, and insurance companies alike—would genuinely want these bills to be correct and accurate. Boy, was I wrong. The slipshod manner in which hospitals and other medical facilities currently bill their patients—and in which insurance carriers pay their claims—seems to profit everybody involved.

Everyone, that is, except for the patient.

What I've found through the years is a system so convoluted that it actually discourages accuracy and encourages error. Just what kinds of errors am I talking about? Consider these examples:

- One Virginia hospital billed a couple for the circumcision of their newborn. Not an unreasonable charge, really, except for the fact that the couple had a baby girl.
- An Illinois hospital billed a man $186,000 for "heart valves." *Two hundred* heart valves, that is.
- Another Virginia hospital billed a patient for the use of its delivery room. Odd, since the man was in the hospital for heart surgery.

What most distresses me about these mistakes is the amount of work it took to uncover them. Had each family involved not rolled up their sleeves and made a concerted effort to investigate their medical bills, they (and probably their insurance carriers too) would have never known what they had paid for!

Many of the problems in health care billing are unintentional, to be sure. Some stem from simple clerical errors keyed in by data-entry workers being paid little more than the minimum wage. Many more problems, however, might rightly be classified as fraud (many already have, as we'll see later).

Whether intentional or not, the problems are endemic. It's the system as a whole that allows and even promotes these errors, and it's the system as a whole that we need to fix if we're ever going to stop the madness you're about to read about.

WHAT TO EXPECT

Many of you reading this aren't all that interested in reforming the system, I know. You just want to find out if *your* medical bills are wrong, and if *you've* paid out—or are about to pay out—money you shouldn't have. That's fine. It's for that reason I wrote this book.

In the pages that follow, we'll take a brief look at how we got into the mess we're in, then we'll help you find your way out. You'll be given tools to help you navigate your way through the murky waters of medical overcharges and mischarges and of wrongful treatment by your insurance company or HMO.

People call me a medical sleuth. That may be the case, but I'll be the first to tell you I haven't any medical background whatsoever.

I first started investigating medical bills more than fifteen years ago when I stumbled upon a $400 overcharge in a bill my father received for a routine medical procedure. Most of what I've learned since then I've learned by self-education, by trial and error, by dogged determination, by luck, and sometimes (I'll admit) by accident. Through the years, though, I have been fortunate to have many top health professionals and consumer advocates lend me their expertise and insights.

You can learn from my experiences.

When I first started getting patients' money back from their medical bills, I had no idea that people weren't already doing this sort of thing all over the country. I thought surely others must be seeing these problems and were busy working to fix them. Apparently, I was wrong again.

I'm confident this book can help you recover money that rightfully belongs to you—money currently in the wrongful possession of hospitals, doctors, insurance companies, and HMOs. At the same time, I hope I open everybody's eyes to the *other* health care crisis in America—the crisis in medical billing. I hope this book forces all Americans to wake up and demand that common sense and courtesy be returned to our health care billing system.

The stakes are tremendously high.

Did you know that we Americans spend more of our gross national product on health care than we do on defense and education *combined?* In any given year, we receive more medical tests, undergo more operations, and take more drugs than much of the world's population ever receive in their lifetime!

In one sense, we enjoy the best health care in the world. Our health care system is second to none in areas such as medical research, drug development, and technological innovation.

Yet in another sense, few would dispute that our health care system really stinks. Medicare fraud has gotten so bad that ordinary drug dealers are scrambling to get in on the action. The rate of medical inflation runs three times higher than the rate of inflation in general. More than thirty-five million Americans have no health insurance to cover the rising costs.

And at the same time, nine out of ten medical bills are just plain wrong!

The way we're expected to pay for our health care has turned into a comedy of errors. It's time we recognize this disease that's afflicting us and put a stop to the nonsense.

However, I need to forewarn you. Even if you read this book from cover to cover and put all the information I share in it to good use, don't fool yourself into thinking you have all the answers to the problems that might beset you. Like passengers standing on the bow of the ill-fated *Titanic,* we're only seeing the tip of a disastrous iceberg.

If I've learned anything over the past fifteen years, it's that for every trick we uncover, two more lie in wait.

2

The Price of
Ignorance

WHY THIS BOOK HAS TO BE READ

On Friday, March 29, 1998, Gary Wahl suffered a severe heart attack. His family and friends were caught completely off guard. He was only thirty-two years old.

In a panic, Gary's wife, Susan, rushed him to the nearest emergency room in their newly adopted hometown of San Diego. He was taken into surgery immediately.

It was successful. Gary survived.

But four days later Susan found herself panicking again. Gary was now ready to be discharged from the hospital, but a woman in the finance department to which Susan had been directed was telling her that if she didn't pay his bill in its entirety on the spot, the hospital couldn't release him.

Couldn't release him?

Susan asked what the total bill came to. "Approximately $7,500," she was told.

Approximately? Susan thought a moment, then asked if this wasn't the final bill. Probably not, the lady said, but it would definitely be the "majority" of the bill. Other minor charges would probably be added to it following discharge, she explained.

Feeling a bit light-headed, Susan asked if the hospital required everyone to pay before they left the hospital. "Yes, we do," she was told. The hospital was well aware that Gary and Susan had no health insurance. Susan asked if some other arrangement might be made. They just didn't have $7,500 lying around.

"Why don't you put it on a credit card?" the lady suggested.

"Any other alternatives?" Susan asked.

Perhaps, Susan was told, but if any further negotiations could be made, they'd have to be made through another person in the finance department. And that guy wasn't available.

"But you can't even tell me if this bill is accurate at this point!" Susan protested.

That's something she'd need to take up with the other guy, too. "Tell you what I can do," the lady continued. "Pay in full right now, and I'll knock 20 percent off the balance."

Not knowing what else to do, Susan handed over her Citibank card.

A few months later, Susan Wahl described to me in a letter her feelings of hurt and betrayal. She said she felt the hospital deliberately tried to take advantage of her during a very distressing and vulnerable time. "The fact that we had no family in San Diego—and that I'd never had the experience of discharging someone from a hospital before—made it all terribly confusing," she said. "Not only did the woman make me feel as though I had to pay off the entire bill right then and there, she even coerced me to do so by offering me a discount!"

Worse than that, Susan felt, she was lied to.

The "minor" charges mentioned by the lady in the finance department? She was right, the charges did appear later. But they were hardly "minor." Susan received two more bills from the hospital—one for an additional $10,000, another for $2,000 more.

"I feel the whole situation was fraudulent," she said.

THE GANG THAT CAN'T BILL STRAIGHT

Extreme as her situation may have been, millions of Americans would probably want to stand up and say *Amen!* to Susan's complaints. Many of us can relate to her feelings of frustration with her local hospital. We've had our own run-ins with our own health care providers' billing departments.

Hospitals in particular have turned into what *Money* magazine has called "the gang that can't bill straight." Within the span of a few short years, medical billing practices have gone from being unquestionable to being unintelligible, from being arrogant to being downright absurd.

How bad has the problem gotten?

Money magazine estimates that consumers are being overcharged to the tune of about $10 billion a year! The U.S. General Accounting Office backs them up.

Pause for just a moment and think about that figure— ten *billion* dollars overcharged *every* year!

How could we have allowed ourselves to get into this

mess? It's a question worth trying to answer. While I'm no economist, I do have some ideas.

A BRIEF HISTORY OF CRIME

Think about it.

A long time ago in a galaxy far, far away, all patients paid their medical bills out of their own pockets. Then, as medical care progressed and grew more expensive, we started paying health insurance companies monthly premiums to pay those high costs for us—if and when we ever needed it. Fortunately, a lot of us never needed it, so insurance companies started growing fat off our premiums.

Health care providers soon realized that all they had to do was tell the insurance companies how much to pay, and they would pay it. Because the insurance companies could pass along the inflated medical costs to their customers through higher premiums, they had no real reason to complain.

Before long, hospitals and other medical facilities enjoyed unprecedented license in pricing their goods and services. The insurance companies just kept paying!

Then things got a little tight for the insurance companies. Competition heated up. Managed care entered the picture. Costs were suddenly being driven down (unnaturally so in the case of many health maintenance organizations).

Insurance companies were forced to stop writing blank checks to the health care providers. Now the providers were in a pickle. More and more, their patients' bills were either being paid by stingy insurance companies or by downright ornery HMOs. A double whammy! Nobody was willing to pay the exaggerated prices anymore.

But the medical community had built its practices upon foundations of exaggerated prices! They had to get the money from *somewhere*.

Their solution?

Build costs into anything and everything the insurance companies and HMOs would still pay a decent wage for. Slip it into the room charge. Slip it into the lab charge. Slip it into the X rays. Slip it into the bedpan. Whatever it took.

And here we are today.

Charges are being slipped to us anywhere and everywhere health care administrators can stick them. Crazy as it sounds, the only people still paying full price to health care facilities are the patients themselves—particularly the uninsured and the poorly insured!

That's right. You and I are picking up the difference between a health care system that *was* and a health care system that *is*.

But, you should be asking yourself, how could we have been so blind? How could we have allowed them to stick it to us so ruthlessly? How could we have let them pull the wool so completely over our eyes? The answer is as simple as it is scary, and it's where we need to begin our quest to right our medical billing wrongs.

THE MAN WHO KNEW TOO MUCH

Unfortunately, hospitals and other medical facilities have learned that the more ignorant their customers are, the less they'll question.

Susan Wahl's experience, though taken to an extreme, was for the most part typical. Before anyone leaves a hospital, they're almost always directed to the finance or admissions office to "set up a payment plan." Often the hospital will pressure people to pay the balance right then and there.

Don't you fall for it. As Susan figured out, more often than not the hospital doesn't even know what the balance is at that point.

I love the story of the man who, like Susan, was told by his hospital that he couldn't take his wife home until he paid her bill. Unlike Susan, though, he'd have none of it. Very calmly the man walked across the lobby to a pay phone and called the local sheriff. "The hospital is holding my wife for ransom," he told him. "I want you to come down here and arrest them for kidnapping." Now there was a man who knew his rights!

The sheriff really did come down. Had the hospital not gone ahead and released her, I'm told the hospital administrator would have been taken into custody.

True story.

Follow his lead. Don't let hospitals or any other health care providers fool you. Don't let them bully you just because you feel you lack the strength, energy, or ability to stand up and fight. Don't let them take advantage of you during a time when you're most vulnerable.

Stop letting your health care providers bluff you into paying for things you don't owe. You should not be made to shoulder the burdens of a health care system that's financially out of whack.

ACTION POINTS

☐ **Wake up!** Times have changed. Hospitals aren't billing straight, and insurers aren't reimbursing straight. You shouldn't allow yourself to get squeezed between a health care system that *was* and a health care system that *is*.

☐ **Refuse to be bullied.** Resolve not to allow yourself to be pressured by any health care provider into paying money you don't owe.

☐ **Refuse to pay as you go.** Don't be duped into believing you have to pay off your bill before you leave the hospital or clinic following a major procedure. Remember, it's much too early for anyone to tell you how much is really owed at this point, much less who's responsible for payment.

3

The Sum of All Fears

WHEN A BILL IS NOT A BILL

The first thing you need to understand is this: We're idiots.

Medical idiots, I mean.

We have entrusted our health care to third and fourth parties for so long, we don't know the first thing about what it is we're paying for when we go to the hospital or doctor.

Believe me, our health care providers know this, *and they use it to their advantage.* One way they do this is through the overt sort of bullying tactics Susan Wahl encountered. Another way they do it is much more covert and, sadly, almost universal in its use. You've no doubt encountered it yourself.

It's called a *summary bill.* And it's the root of all kinds of evil.

Health care facilities don't as a matter of practice send

out itemized bills like other businesses in other industries do. They send out summary bills. You need to know the difference.

An itemized hospital bill can run ten to twenty to two-hundred-plus pages long. A summary bill is almost always one page.

If you've ever been treated at a hospital, I can almost guarantee you were sent a summary bill, not an itemized bill. The statement you were given told you what to pay but not what you were paying for.

Most people never notice the difference.

Why not? Two reasons, I think.

First, most of us have some type of insurance paying the bulk of our bills. We figure, why waste time scrutinizing a bill that somebody else is taking care of? We assume that our insurance company, since they're picking up more of the tab than we are, would surely cry foul if they detected any mistakes or irregularities. Surely they're checking. And surely they know more about this sort of thing than we ever could.

Wrong. Wrong. And wrong again.

Insurance companies have neither the time nor the resources to scrutinize each individual claim that's filed. Sure, they have audit departments, but their auditing can only go so far. Only in the most unusual of circumstances will they ever go so far as to order and examine someone's medical charts to make sure that what's on the bill actually matches the claim. The primary concern of insurance company auditors is just to make sure that all the treatments billed are appropriate to the illness or injury being treated.

And that's it.

The second reason most people never notice that their medical bill is summarized and not itemized is that the summary bill actually *looks* like a regular bill. While it doesn't itemize the goods and services you received, it does (in the case of a hospital) break down your bill into six or seven *categories* of charges: room, pharmacy, laboratory, medical/surgical supplies, and that sort of thing.

In other words, it *looks* as if it's itemized. It *looks* accurate.

Wrong again.

Take a look at the following example of a hospital summary bill (figure 3a). Then look at just a few pages of the very same bill *itemized* (figure 3b).

If the total dollar amount of each category on the first bill always matched up with the sum of all the *itemized* charges for each category found on the second bill, that would make the summary bill appear accurate. The totals often do add up accurately (not always, but often).

And yet, nine out of ten medical bills are still wrong.

The problems, unfortunately, are usually buried a little deeper. They begin to surface only when one takes the time to see what each of the itemized charges actually is.

You've probably heard it said that God is in the details. That may well be true for architecture and other pursuits, but in the case of medical billing, fools have rushed in where angels have feared to tread. If anybody, it's the devil who's in the details!

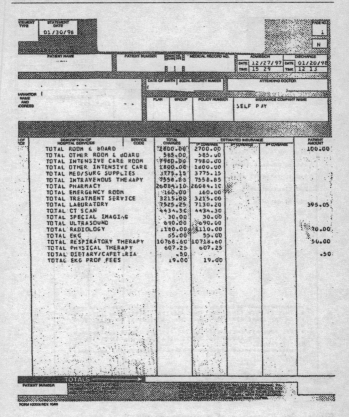

Figure 3a: Example of a summary bill

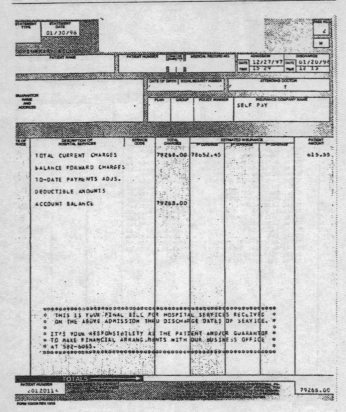

Figure 3a: Example of a summary bill

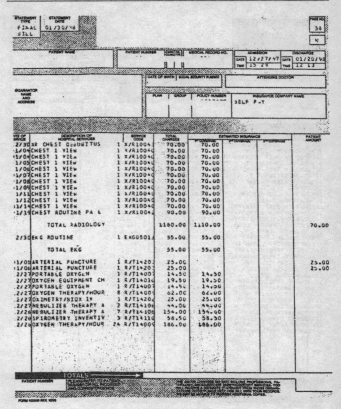

Figure 3b: Example of an itemized bill

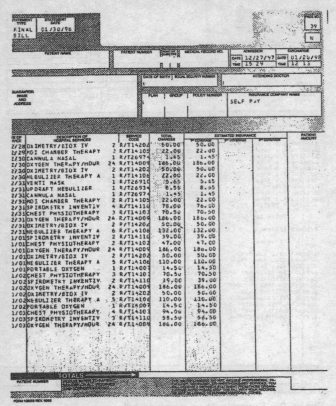

Figure 3b: Example of an itemized bill

Think of it this way: What if the next time you go to your local grocery store the clerk hands you a receipt that looks like this?

```
DEWEY CHEATUM
SUPERMARKET

Produce          $31.66
Meats            $26.54
Dairy            $18.07
Toiletries       $25.81
Dry Goods        $39.95
Miscellaneous   $210.75
Subtotal        $352.78
Tax              $17.64
TOTAL           $370.42


Thank You for
Shopping Dewey
Cheatum!
Have A Nice Day!
```

Would you go back to a supermarket that billed you like this?

I know *I* wouldn't.

If you're like me, every time you buy groceries you probably read through the register tape on the way out the door, or in the car, or as you put away your food once you get home.

Why do we do this?

Because we want to know if the scanner at the check-out counter scanned each item correctly. We want to know if the clerk counted six cans of soup when we only bought four. We want to make sure the computer figured in that specially advertised price on milk.

We want to make sure we got exactly what we paid for, right?

Of course.

The following grocery receipt is the way receipts are supposed to look. You buy something, it shows up on the bill in recognizable form along with a recognizable price.

HAPPY VALLEY SUPERMARKET 6/21/2000		Deodorant	$2.39
		Peppers	$ .89
		Potatoes	$1.08
		Newspaper	$1.50
Tomatoes	$1.54	Salsa	$2.69
Cucumbers	$ .99	Chips	$2.99
Cheese	$1.69	Pasta	$1.09
Broccoli	$1.39	Macaroni	$ .79
Lettuce	$1.19	Milk	$1.69
Bananas	$1.34	Juice	$2.19
Eggs	$1.49	Cola	$1.99
Yogurt	$2.19	Subtotal	$32.78
Bread	$1.89	Tax	$ 1.70
Onions	$ .59	TOTAL	$34.48
Cookies	$2.29		
Hot Dogs	$2.99	Thank You for	
Buns	$ .89	Shopping at	
Bagels	$2.19	Happy Valley.	
Carrots	$ .69	Have A Nice Day!	

Now *that's* an itemized bill: one that tells us exactly what we've paid for.

We expect our supermarkets to itemize each of our purchases. We expect our drugstores to itemize each of our purchases. We expect our department stores, hardware stores, and restaurants to do the same.

Why don't we expect the same from our hospitals?

The summary bill is the hospital's best attempt to get you to pay an unknown sum.

Don't fall for it. Tell them to send you an itemized bill instead.

Here's the thing: *They have to do it*. Every state now requires by law its health care facilities to provide patients itemized accounts of the charges they have incurred—if and when the patient asks for one.

So all you have to do is ask for it!

But even with the law on your side, be prepared to catch some flack when you ask.

SEVEN HABITS OF HIGHLY DEFLECTIVE PEOPLE

Health care facilities, and hospitals in particular, have developed some tried-and-true tactics to help them avoid giving out itemized statements, and they're never shy in using them. If you request an itemization, be prepared to hear a variation on one of the following themes:

1) The "What's up, Doc?" ("An itemized statement? Why would you want that?") As if you must be from Mars to make such an odd request.

Your answer: "I'd simply like to know what I'm really paying for. Is that a problem?"

2) The raised eyebrow. ("And just *why* do you want one of *those*?") Do they think you're just trying to make trouble for the kindly folks who have worked so hard to heal you?

Your answer: "I don't pay for anything sight unseen. Is that a problem?"

3) The artful dodge. ("Oh, don't worry about it—your insurance is paying it.") After all, why should you care about things like insurance and your health?

Your answer: "Maybe so. But should they refuse to cover something—which, as *you* know, they're doing more and more these days—I'll need to be informed as well."

4) The fear of God. ("We've already sent your bill over to collections. You'll have to try and get it from them.") *This* one sounds to me like you'll incur further bodily harm should you push the issue.

Your answer: "I understand that for a request such as this the collection agency will just send me right back to you. Isn't that true?"

5) The bald-faced lie. ("You can't get one." Or, if you've already paid the bill but want to go back and check it: "Since it's already paid for, you can't receive one.") When did it become a physical impossibility to print out a few computer pages?

Your answer: "I know that state law requires that you give me an itemized statement. I also know that it doesn't matter whether I've paid it or not, you're required to provide me with one."

6) The strong arm. ("We consider that kind of request an 'intent to audit.' Ninety percent of the bill must be paid before we can begin an audit.") They actually do say that— as if they have you on a legal technicality!

Your answer: "Nonsense. I don't intend to audit anything. I just want to see what it is you're asking me to pay for. You and I both know you're required by law to provide me with an itemized bill. I'd really rather not, but do I need to call my lawyer?"

If after giving you one or two excuses a billing clerk still refuses to give you an itemized bill, then politely ask to speak with the financial director. That request alone should get you your actual bill.

But even then—even after the billing department agrees to send you an itemized bill—don't be surprised if you run into:

7) The classic. ("It's in the mail.")

Your answer: "I really can't wait. Could you please just print me off a copy while I'm here?" Or, if you happen to be calling by phone: "Let me just drop by and pick up a copy, okay?"

Think I'm kidding?

A 1998 study on hospital billing published in the research journal *Organizational Science* backs my experience up with "clinical data." The article claims that the hospitals in the study "promoted anticipatory, bureaucratic images by presenting *bureaucratic roadblocks* to patients who questioned their bill or challenged charges. These roadblocks were not responses to specific questions, but detours that prevented patients from getting information that may have escalated their questions."

Roadblocks and detours. Sound familiar?

The authors of the study call such tactics "anticipatory impression management," even "anticipatory obfuscation." The study quotes various hospital representatives—billing clerks—telling how and why they avoid giving out itemized bills:

- "I'll tell them to go after their insurance company if they are dissatisfied because my hands are tied," said one.

- "I say charges are normal and customary," said another. "I don't try to explain individual charges. I just say that over and over until they get tired of hearing it."

- One group of representatives said they purposely avoid coughing up itemized bills because "patients can't understand them and they cause more questions."

- Another representative stated outright that part of her job was to prevent patients from "moving up the ladder with questions."

Frustrated patients quoted in the study also concur:

- Patient #1: "I tried to talk about [the bill] with the billing office, and I said I don't understand these charges. They weren't helpful, they were reading the insurance policy to me, and I said, well I read it, and they said then you should have understood that this says customary charges. To all my questions they would open the insurance policy and read from it. So they sort of skirted the issue completely, as far as explaining charges. They were very bureaucratic. There was a young woman there, and she kind of made me feel like I was bothering her. I think I stopped asking after a couple of questions. I felt kind of helpless. I wanted to do something. but I didn't know what to do. So I decided I better start paying $100 a month just in case."

- Patient #2: "You know it wasn't going to make any difference. You know you could beat your head against the wall some more, but in the long run it really wasn't going to make a big difference. So you just pay."

You just pay.

IT'S UP TO YOU

For years, doctors have been urging us to take control of our own health care through preventive measures such as exercise, diet, and right living. That's great advice. In the same way, it's time we take control of our health care *finances*—through preventive measures such as due diligence and common sense. Assuming responsibility for the accuracy of your medical bills is right living too.

Even those of us with "good" insurance coverage can't afford to live with the false notion that our insurance companies are guarding our financial interests. As I said earlier, they can't, and they're not. They lack both the resources and the know-how.

Remember, even if your insurance policy covers 100 percent of your medical expenses, which I doubt it does, you'll still get stuck footing the bill through higher deductibles and premiums. (Not to mention that there'll almost surely be some discomforting surprises waiting for you in the language of your insurance policy itself, as we'll discuss in later chapters.)

If for some reason you feel you just can't get a handle on your own medical bills, then get someone to do it for you. Appendix B contains a list of companies that can help you, many of which charge on a contingency basis only.

Oh, yes. One other thing . . . The bills that hospitals and some other providers (such as long-term care facilities) send out—even once they've been itemized—still probably won't be, shall we say, *all-inclusive*. If you've been hospitalized any length of time at all, you'll probably start getting bills from doctors and offices you'll swear you never heard of before!

Many of the doctors who treat you at the hospital, for instance—whether they remove your gall bladder or just pop their head into the door to ask how you're feeling—will bill you separately. That's because most of the doctors who work *at* a hospital don't work *for* the hospital. They work for themselves and their own private practices. But they too like to send summary bills.

We'll talk more about them later, but remember, the same rules apply. Get the bills itemized.

ACTION POINTS

❏ **Get a real bill.** Recognize the difference between a summary bill and an itemized bill. Should your hospital or doctor send you a summary bill with only categories of charges listed (which they probably will), ask them also to give you an itemized bill that details every specific expense you have incurred.

❏ **Refuse to take no for an answer.** Should a hospital or doctor in any way try to avoid giving you an itemized bill, remind them politely yet firmly that they must do so under penalty of state law. Tell them that no matter how strange a request they think it is, no matter how much insurance you have, no matter where the bill has been "sent," no matter how little or how much you've already paid, they are required to give you an itemized bill. Ask to talk to a manager when necessary.

❏ **Keep itemizing.** Also get itemized bills from any health care professionals who happen to bill you separately following a major medical procedure.

❏ **Take control.** Remember that the only person watching out for your interests is *you*—not your hospital, not your doctor, and not your insurance carrier or health maintenance organization.

❏ **If necessary, get help.** Find someone to review your bills for you if you cannot or do not want to do so yourself.

4

Greek 101
HOW YOU CAN LEARN THEIR LANGUAGE

There's an old episode of *The Andy Griffith Show* in which Sheriff Andy Taylor and his comical sidekick, Deputy Barney Fife, follow a suspected jewel thief away from their hometown of Mayberry, North Carolina, to the fictional "big town" of Mount Pilot. Their undercover surveillance leads them to dine one evening in a fancy French restaurant.

Andy, looking down at the menu and realizing that all the items are written in French, turns to the waiter and asks him, "Can I just have a steak?"

The waiter isn't impressed, but he takes the order nonetheless.

Barney, on the other hand, too proud to let his lack of sophistication show, tries to suavely select his dinner without saying a word. "I'll have *that*," he says, directing the waiter's attention to an item on the menu. "And *that*," he says smugly, adding another item to his order.

When the food arrives, Sheriff Taylor gets exactly what he ordered, as does Deputy Fife. But while Andy is satisfied, Barney is stunned.

It turns out that Barney Fife had unwittingly ordered brains and snails.

The moral of this little story is simply this: If you don't know what something means, don't be afraid to ask!

Whether you're talking with a waiter in a fancy French restaurant or with the head of medical records at your local hospital, the principle is still the same. Don't be intimidated. It's far better to admit your ignorance and get your steak than it is to act like you know something you really don't and get "slugged" instead.

GREEK TO YOU AND ME

Off the top of my head, I can't think of any hospital in the United States whose medical records are written in French. But I do know far too many who write—and sometimes speak!—in Greek.

At least that's the way it sounds to you and me.

If you don't know what I'm talking about, take a look at your itemized bill. If yours is anything like the one you saw in the last chapter (and unfortunately for you, it is), it too has nonsensical words and phrases like "STOPCOCK, 3-WAY, OMX-234" and "CHEM 8" and "D5%/LACTATED RINGERS 1000ML" and "TRAY TPN CVP SUBCLAVIAN."

Like I said, "Greek."

In fact, if you're anything like me, your first thoughts upon seeing an itemized hospital bill might have been: *RUN*

AWAY! Forget this nonsense! Take me back to the summary bill! I'd rather just pay whatever they ask than try to decode this stuff!

I understand. I was there too.

But it's not nearly as bad as it looks, as long as you have help. You don't even need to learn to speak Greek. You just need to be able to translate the medical codes, terms, and abbreviations that hinder your understanding of the goods and services you're paying for. And for that, all you really need to do is find the right people to ask and the right "Greek-to-English dictionaries" to refer to.

Is this necessary? Yes.

If we're to survive and conquer our medical bills, there's just no way around it: We need to learn enough of their language to recognize the errors those bills contain. It's up to *us* to overcome the language barrier between our common, everyday English and their less-than-ordinary "medicalspeak."

After all, how can we possibly expect to fix errors we can't spot?

IN THEIR DEFENSE

There is, of course, a bona fide reason why itemized medical bills and other medical records are unintelligible to the untrained eye. With no common language, there could be no effective continuum of care from coast to coast. And if they couldn't use shorthand (codes and abbreviations and such), then our doctors, nurses, and therapists would find themselves even further awash in the paperwork that's already drowning them.

The medical community nationwide needs a common

vocabulary for its members to be able to deal with one another effectively and efficiently. It's absolutely critical that a long-term care facility in Walla Walla be able to read the medical chart accompanying a new resident from Washington, D.C. Likewise, it's crucial that a pharmacist in Charlotte be able to fill prescriptions written by doctors in Chicago and Cheyenne.

Because it's important that the medical community's language be extremely accurate and specific (remember, lives *are* at stake), the use of technical jargon—as strange as it may sound to our nontechnical ears—is a necessary evil. And because it's important for doctors and nurses to be able to write and read quickly, the use of medical shorthand—both numeric codes and simple abbreviations—is necessary too.

We can't fault the medical community for speaking Greek. But neither can we ignore their conversation just because it sounds a little foreign to our ears.

THE PAPER CHASE

Our task is simple, though not easy: We need to decipher the gibberish that's written on our itemized bill and then match it to the gibberish that's written in our medical records.

That's it.

In a nutshell, *that* is how you right your medical bill's wrongs. Simple, but rarely easy.

You've gotten your itemized bill. Now you need to get your medical records.

How do you get them? All it takes is a brief, written request to your hospital's medical records department, which keeps a file on you containing every medical-related jot and tittle recorded during your stay.

Your request needs only to contain a few bits of information: your name, your signature and Social Security number; the date of your hospitalization; and where you want the records sent. (If you want your medical records released to a third party—such as a medical billing advocate who's helping you navigate your way through your medical bills—feel free. The records don't have to go directly to you.)

You can use this sample format for your request:

August 1, 2000

Medical Records
Acme Medical Center
1 Long Road
Anytown, US 12345

Dear Medical Records:

Please promptly forward a copy of all medical records pertaining to my hospitalization of July 4–8, 2000 to:

> Jane Doe
> 21 Maple Street
> Anytown, US 12345

Thank you for your help,
Jane Doe
SS# 123-45-6789

All it takes is this little letter . . . and maybe $150. *Say again?*

You heard me right. I wish I was kidding, but the truth is many hospitals will stick you for *photocopying* charges. (The hospital has to keep the original records on file, of course.) I've seen hospitals charge anywhere from 10 cents to $2.75 per page.

Most hospitals add to that charge a "retrieval fee" of about $10 to cover searching, handling, and mailing.

Do the math. In the case of a prolonged hospital stay or one involving multiple procedures, you might have amassed a couple hundred pages of medical records. At a dollar per page, that adds up to . . . serious cash!

A significant number of states (twenty at present) have statutes that limit the amount of money their hospitals can charge for copying fees. In my home state of Virginia, for instance, hospitals can charge up to 50 cents per page for the first fifty pages, then 25 cents for every page thereafter. In California and Colorado they can only charge up to 25 cents, period (with a minimum request of $10 in Colorado).

In the state of Florida, though, hospitals can and do charge up to one dollar per page. On the opposite end of the spectrum, Kentucky is the only state whose hospitals are mandated by law to send you your first set of medical records free of charge.

Ironically, almost every hospital in America outsources their medical record copying to one of three or so national companies. My experience has been that while these companies undoubtedly know the state laws limiting what they can charge, they don't care to follow them. So you need to know the law in your state. (The American Health Information Management Association lists online the amount each state allows at http://www.ahima.org/publications/2a/pract.brief.0199a.html.)

In most cases, thankfully, the copying fees are manageable. Unfortunately, if your hospital is within its rights to charge you a buck or two per page, the most you can do is cry foul to your local legislator.

The truth of the matter is we *all* need to cry foul to our local legislators. I believe *every* state should follow Kentucky's lead. Every state ought to mandate its hospitals to give patients at least one copy of their medical records free of charge upon request. That's not just common sense, that's common decency.

If a patient has requested these records to review them for errors, and he or she does in fact find errors in them, shouldn't the hospital cover the copying costs, regardless of the number of copies made?

Until we get to that commonsense point, so as not to waste your time, it's important that you call your medical records department to determine any fees they may charge *before* you send in your written request.

But photocopying fees notwithstanding, getting your medical records from your hospital should *not* be a major ordeal.

CHARTING YOUR COURSE

When you do get your medical records, what exactly will you find?

Depending on the nature of your illness or injury, these are specific records you might receive from your hospital's medical records department:

History and Physical   Discusses your perti-
                                  nent medical history
                                  and the specific reason

why you were admitted
to the hospital.

Discharge Summary

Summarizes your entire
hospital stay.

Physician's Orders

Documents all the sup-
plies, medications, lab
work, and treatments
your doctor ordered for
you.

Physician's Progress Notes

Contains daily notes
written by your doctors,
describing your progress
as a patient.

Nursing Notes

Discusses your progress,
treatments, and daily
activities from the eyes
of the nurses who at-
tended to your care.

Nursing Medication Sheet

Documents what med-
ications you actually
took.

Operating Report

Contains the detailed
report of a surgical pro-
cedure you underwent.

Recovery Room Report

Documents the services
you received while you
were recuperating in the
recovery room following
surgery.

Anesthesia Report	Documents the services performed by the anesthesiologist.
Emergency Room Report	Documents all services performed for you in the ER.
Laboratory Report	Documents all laboratory tests, services, and procedures.
X-Ray Report	Indicates the results of any X rays taken.
Therapy Notes	Documents all services provided by physical, occupational, speech, and respiratory therapists.

Different hospitals occasionally have different names for some of these records. For instance, your hospital might send you a "Flow Sheet" in lieu of "Nursing Notes." Regardless of the title of the record, the pertinent information should still be there.

If you happen to find some pages missing (say, one particular date), which happens from time to time, call the medical records department and have them find those records and send them to you.

KENTUCKY FRIED CHICKEN SCRATCH

Once you have your medical records in hand, you now find yourself faced with one of modern science's few remaining riddles: doctors' handwriting.

Frightening, no?

Compounding the problem of simple bad handwriting is the fact that doctors' orders are usually chock-full of abbreviations, symbols, and codes. Ideally, this medical shorthand should be universally understood by all, making the reading of these charts easier and more convenient.

The reality, however, is that the medical community has a common language with many different dialects.

To an extent, this is to be expected. Surgeons will write and speak differently from psychiatrists, who will write and speak differently from pharmacists, who will write and speak differently from physical therapists. While there will be some universal understanding among all of them, each field within medical care has its own terminology, complete with its own interpretations.

Take the simple abbreviation "OD," for instance.

Most of us recognize this as an abbreviation for the word *overdose* (as in "the fifty-six-year-old rock star *OD'd* on heroin and was rushed to the nearest hospital, along with his twenty-one-year-old girlfriend.") And so it's used within the medical community.

But that's not the *only* way it's used within the medical community.

The abbreviation "OD" might also mean "once daily," as in the case of a doctor's instructions to a nurse: "This medication is to be taken once daily."

An ophthalmologist, meanwhile, might write down the letters "OD" to refer to the patient's "right eye" when he's conducting an eye exam!

Another common abbreviation used by the medical community is the letter "U." More often than not, the letter "U" refers to "units." But "U" could also mean "urine." Or "upper." Or it might just mean "unknown."

There are many other such examples—for instance, "DC" can mean "discharge" or "discontinue," "PO" can mean "postoperative" or "by mouth"—but you get the picture.

Does it matter that abbreviations like "OD" and "U" can refer to three or four entirely different things?

Clearly, it matters when an abbreviation is misinterpreted by medical personnel, which happens. I confess I've not come across too many patients who've had an aspirin administered in their "right eye" when they were supposed to have taken it "once daily"! But in a recent *Reader's Digest* article, C. Everett Koop, former surgeon general of the United States, warned readers, "Deciphering a doctor's scribbled handwriting, a busy pharmacist could mistake Norvasc, a calcium channel blocker, for Navane, used to treat psychotic disorders. Cerebyx, an anti-convulsant, might be confused with Celebrex, an anti-inflammatory drug, or Celexa, an anti-depressant."

It definitely matters, then.

Abbreviations—which are intended to speed up the paperwork process—can actually slow our medical care down. When nurses have to read and then reread a chart to make sure that they're interpreting the doctors' orders correctly, it obviously delays the care that the patient is supposed to be receiving.

For our present purposes, the confusion really matters when *you* are staring at a medical chart that looks like the example on page 45, and you're trying to match the gibberish on it to the gibberish on your itemized bill.

Neil Davis, a professor at the Temple University School of Pharmacy, has self-published a little book called *Medical Abbreviations* that can be of great benefit to anyone trying to decode such shorthand. It's inexpensive and can save you invaluable time and frustration.

Example of physician's orders sheet

Davis has compiled 14,000 abbreviations into one volume. Still, as he states in the foreword to the book, these represent only a portion of the abbreviations currently in use.

You may have to have your local bookstore special-order it for you, but I highly recommend it. (You can order it directly from the publisher at: Neil M. Davis Associates, 1143 Wright Drive, Huntington, PA 19006.)

Example of physician's progress notes

BLACK CODES FROM THE UNDERGROUND

Getting back to your itemized medical bill, let's take a look at a different sort of medical abbreviation. These are the abbreviations and codes that, even though typed neatly, still read like chicken scratch. These are the "STOPCOCK, 3-WAY, OMX-234" and the "CHEM 8" and the "D5%/LACTATED RINGERS 1000ML" and the "TRAY TPN CVP SUBCLAVIAN."

INPATIENT STATEMENT OF ACCOUNT

PATIENT NAME	ACCOUNT NO.	ADMISSION DATE	DISCHARGE DATE	STATEMENT DATE
		09/02/94	09/14/94	09/17/94

PLEASE REFER TO PATIENT'S NAME AND ACCOUNT NO. ON ALL CORRESPONDENCE.

DATE DUE ▶

▶ PAY THIS AMOUNT ◀

Make check payable to: BENTARA HOSPITALS

PLEASE SHOW
AMOUNT PAID ⟶ $

TO ENSURE PROPER CREDIT - DETACH AND RETURN TOP PORTION OF THIS STATEMENT WITH PAYMENT. DO NOT FOLD OR STAPLE.

PATIENT NAME		ACCOUNT NO.		INSURANCE PORTION IS COMPUTED ACCORDING TO THE INFORMATION SUPPLIED BY YOUR INSURANCE CARRIER.	STATEMENT DATE	PAGE NO.
		...			09/17/94	01

SERVICE DATE	REF. NO.	DESCRIPTION	TOTAL AMOUNT	EST. INSURANCE	PATIENT PORTION
		— SUMMARY OF CHARGES —			
		— ROOM CHARGES —			
	001	PRIVATE			
		12 DAYS AT 215.00	2580.00	2580.00	
		TOTAL OF ROOM CHARGES	2580.00	2580.00	
		— ANCILLARY CHARGES —			
	230	NURSING ACUITY	1210.00	1210.00	
	250	PHARMACY	3306.50	3306.50	
	260	IV THERAPY	36.20	36.20	
	270	MEDICAL SUPPLIES	1490.78	1490.78	
	300	LAB	1266.00	1266.00	
	312	PATH LAB/CYTOLOGY	210.00	210.00	
	320	X-RAY	88.00	88.00	
	350	CT SCAN	1260.00	1260.00	
	360	OPERATING ROOM	1302.93	1302.93	
	370	ANESTHESIA	610.14	610.14	
	400	DIAGNOSTIC SERVICES	253.00	253.00	
	410	RESPIRATORY SERVICES	342.47	342.47	
	450	EMERGENCY ROOM	239.00	239.00	
	710	RECOVERY ROOM	550.35	550.35	
	730	EKG/ECG	64.73	64.73	

WE HAVE FILED THE FOLLOWING INSURANCE
BLUE CROSS KEYCARE
INSURANCE BENEFITS ASSIGNED ▶

PATIENT PLEASE PAY
DUE & PAYABLE UPON RECEIPT.

THESE CHARGES DO NOT INCLUDE FEES FOR PROFESSIONAL SERVICES RENDERED. YOU WILL RECEIVE A SEPARATE BILL FROM THE PHYSICIAN.

PLEASE EXAMINE THIS STATEMENT CAREFULLY. THIS WILL BE YOUR ONLY ITEMIZED STATEMENT FOR THE ABOVE TRANSACTIONS. IF YOU HAVE ANY QUESTIONS CONCERNING THIS STATEMENT PLEASE CONTACT ▶ PATIENT ACCOUNTS   Phone:

Example of a summary bill

And the "POT PHOSPHATE 4.4MEQ/MLINJ15ML."
How do you figure out what these mean?
Ask.

Call your nurse, call your doctor, call the hospital accounting department. Call whomever you need to find out the meanings behind the abbreviations. Remember, even if

INPATIENT STATEMENT OF ACCOUNT

PATIENT NAME	ACCOUNT NO.	ADMISSION DATE	DISCHARGE DATE	STATEMENT DATE
		09/02/94	09/14/94	09/17/94

PLEASE REFER TO PATIENT'S NAME AND ACCOUNT NO. ON ALL CORRESPONDENCE.

DATE DUE ▶ 10/02/94

PAY THIS AMOUNT ▶ 2.75

Make check payable to: SENTARA HOSPITALS

PLEASE SHOW
AMOUNT PAID → $

! TO ENSURE PROPER CREDIT – DETACH AND RETURN TOP PORTION OF THIS STATEMENT WITH PAYMENT. DO NOT FOLD OR STAPLE.

PATIENT NAME	ACCOUNT NO.	INSURANCE PORTION IS COMPUTED ACCORDING TO THE INFORMATION SUPPLIED BY YOUR INSURANCE CARRIER.	STATEMENT DATE	PAGE NO.
			09/17/94	02

SERVICE DATE	REF. NO.	DESCRIPTION	TOTAL AMOUNT	EST. INSURANCE	PATIENT PORTION
	770	PT CONVENIENCE	2.75		2.75
	101	ooo UNKNOWN ooo	218.00	218.00	
		TOTAL CHARGES	15032.85	15030.10	2.75
		PATIENT PAYMENTS	300.00-		300.00
		DEDUCTIBLE & COINSURANCE		300.00-	300.00
		GRAND TOTAL	14732.85	14730.10	

WE HAVE FILED THE FOLLOWING INSURANCE
BLUE CROSS KEYCARE
INSURANCE BENEFITS ASSIGNED ▶

PATIENT
PLEASE PAY ▶   2.75

DUE & PAYABLE UPON RECEIPT.

THESE CHARGES DO NOT INCLUDE FEES FOR
PROFESSIONAL SERVICES RENDERED.
YOU WILL RECEIVE A SEPARATE BILL FROM
THE PHYSICIAN.

PLEASE EXAMINE THIS STATEMENT CAREFULLY. THIS WILL BE YOUR ONLY ITEMIZED STATEMENT FOR THE ABOVE TRANSACTIONS.
IF YOU HAVE ANY QUESTIONS CONCERNING ▶ PATIENT ACCOUNTS   Phone

Example of a summary bill

they're less than enthusiastic to answer your questions, it's better that you get your steak than get "slugged" by your ignorance.

For instance, once I saw a charge on a medical bill for what turned out to be twelve pairs of latex surgical gloves. I called the surgeon directly and asked him just how many

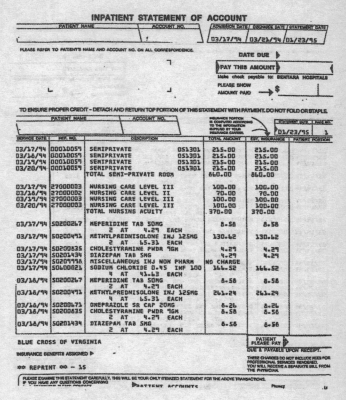

Example of an itemized bill

people had been in the operating room during that surgery. He told me there had been five people present.

So why the extra seven pairs of gloves on the bill? The hospital couldn't justify them. They deducted the charges.

I found out later that the surgeon got his hands slapped by hospital administration for giving me this information!

INPATIENT STATEMENT OF ACCOUNT

PATIENT NAME	ACCOUNT NO.	ADMISSION DATE	DISCHARGE DATE	STATEMENT DATE
		03/17/94	03/21/94	01/23/95

PLEASE REFER TO PATIENT'S NAME AND ACCOUNT NO. ON ALL CORRESPONDENCE.

DATE DUE ▶

▶ PAY THIS AMOUNT

Make check payable to: SENTARA HOSPITALS

PLEASE SHOW
AMOUNT PAID ──▶ $

TO ENSURE PROPER CREDIT – DETACH AND RETURN TOP PORTION OF THIS STATEMENT WITH PAYMENT. DO NOT FOLD OR STAPLE.

PATIENT NAME		ACCOUNT NO.		INSURANCE PORTION IS COMPUTED ACCORDING TO THE INFORMATION SUPPLIED BY YOUR INSURANCE CARRIER	STATEMENT DATE 01/23/95	PAGE NO. 2

SERVICE DATE	REF. NO.	DESCRIPTION	TOTAL AMOUNT	EST. INSURANCE	PATIENT PORTION
03/18/94	50209998	MISCELLANEOUS INJ NON PHARM	NO CHARGE		
03/18/94	50L00021	SODIUM CHLORIDE 0.45 INF 100	41.63	41.63	
03/19/94	50200035	PROCHLORPERAZINE INJ 10MG/2ML	28.66	28.66	
		2 AT 14.33 EACH			
03/19/94	50200047	PREDNISONE TAB 20MG	8.58	8.58	
		2 AT 4.29 EACH			
03/19/94	50200267	MEPERIDINE TAB 50MG	12.87	12.87	
		3 AT 4.29 EACH			
03/19/94	50200335	ESTROGENS CONJ TAB 0.625MG	4.29	4.29	
03/19/94	50200466	SODIUM CHLORIDE 0.9 INJ 2.5M	28.52	28.52	
		2 AT 14.26 EACH			
03/19/94	50200491	METHYLPREDNISOLONE INJ 125MG	130.62	130.62	
		2 AT 65.31 EACH			
03/19/94	50200511	TEMAZEPAM CAP 15MG	5.68	5.68	
		2 AT 2.84 EACH			
03/19/94	50200671	OMEPRAZOLE SR CAP 20MG	8.26	8.26	
03/19/94	50200835	CHOLESTYRAMINE PWDR 9GM	8.58	8.58	
		2 AT 4.29 EACH			
03/19/94	50201250	ALBUTEROL INH 17GM	28.77	28.77	
03/19/94	50201434	DIAZEPAM TAB 5MG	12.87	12.87	
		3 AT 4.29 EACH			
03/19/94	50209998	MISCELLANEOUS INJ NON PHARM	NO CHARGE		
03/20/94	50200035	PROCHLORPERAZINE INJ 10MG/2ML	14.33	14.33	
03/20/94	50200047	PREDNISONE TAB 20MG	8.58	8.58	
		2 AT 4.29 EACH			
03/20/94	50200081	DOXYCYCLINE TAB 100MG	8.45	8.45	
03/20/94	50200267	MEPERIDINE TAB 50MG	8.58	8.58	
		2 AT 4.29 EACH			
03/20/94	50200466	SODIUM CHLORIDE 0.9 INJ 2.5M	42.78	42.78	
		3 AT 14.26 EACH			

BLUE CROSS OF VIRGINIA

INSURANCE BENEFITS ASSIGNED ▶

∞ REPRINT ∞ – 15

PATIENT PLEASE PAY ▶
DUE & PAYABLE UPON RECEIPT.

THESE CHARGES DO NOT INCLUDE FEES FOR PROFESSIONAL SERVICES RENDERED. YOU WILL RECEIVE A SEPARATE BILL FROM THE PHYSICIAN.

PLEASE EXAMINE THIS STATEMENT CAREFULLY. THIS WILL BE YOUR ONLY ITEMIZED STATEMENT FOR THE ABOVE TRANSACTIONS. IF YOU HAVE ANY QUESTIONS CONCERNING

▶ PATIENT ACCOUNTS   Phone)

Example of an itemized bill

Nonetheless, he was glad to help, and my client was glad not to pay for seven pairs of gloves that had no business being on her bill.

Very often you can find the answers you're looking for yourself in a medical dictionary or encyclopedia. In the

INPATIENT STATEMENT OF ACCOUNT

PATIENT NAME	ACCOUNT NO.	ADMISSION DATE	DISCHARGE DATE	STATEMENT DATE
		03/17/94	03/21/94	01/23/95

PLEASE REFER TO PATIENT'S NAME AND ACCOUNT NO. ON ALL CORRESPONDENCE.

DATE DUE ▶

▶PAY THIS AMOUNT

Make check payable to: SENTARA HOSPITALS

PLEASE SHOW

AMOUNT PAID ➡ $

TO ENSURE PROPER CREDIT – DETACH AND RETURN TOP PORTION OF THIS STATEMENT WITH PAYMENT. DO NOT FOLD OR STAPLE.

PATIENT NAME	ACCOUNT NO.

INSURANCE PORTION IS COMPUTED ACCORDING TO THE INFORMATION SUPPLIED BY YOUR INSURANCE CARRIER.

STATEMENT DATE	PAGE NO.
01/23/95	3

SERVICE DATE	REF. NO.	DESCRIPTION	TOTAL AMOUNT	EST. INSURANCE	PATIENT PORTION
03/20/94	50200511	TEMAZEPAM CAP 15MG	5.68	5.68	
		2 AT 2.84 EACH			
03/20/94	50200671	OMEPRAZOLE SR CAP 20MG	8.26	8.26	
03/20/94	50200835	CHOLESTYRAMINE PWDR 9GM	8.58	8.58	
03/20/94	50201434	DIAZEPAM TAB 5MG	8.58	8.58	
		2 AT 4.29 EACH			
03/21/94	50200035	PROCHLORPERAZINE INJ 10MG/2ML	14.33	14.33	
03/21/94	50200047	PREDNISONE TAB 20MG	4.29	4.29	
03/21/94	50200081	DOXYCYCLINE TAB 100MG	8.45	8.45	
03/21/94	50200267	MEPERIDINE TAB 50MG	4.29	4.29	
03/21/94	50200335	ESTROGENS CONJ TAB 0.625MG	4.29	4.29	
03/21/94	50200415	TRIAMCINOLONE INH 60MG/20GM	21.36	21.36	
03/21/94	50200466	SODIUM CHLORIDE 0.9 INJ 2.5M	14.26	14.26	
03/21/94	50200671	OMEPRAZOLE SR CAP 20MG	8.26	8.26	
03/21/94	50200835	CHOLESTYRAMINE PWDR 9GM	8.29	8.29	
03/21/94	50201434	DIAZEPAM TAB 5MG	8.58	8.58	
		2 AT 4.29 EACH			
		TOTAL PHARMACY	1135.09	1135.09	
03/17/94	26000042	IV START	7.00	7.00	
03/19/94	27000043	IV RESTART/TUBING/DSG CHANGE	5.55	5.55	
		TOTAL IV THERAPY	12.55	12.55	
03/17/94	20800006	SPECIMEN COLLECT VENI	16.24	16.24	
		2 AT 8.12 EACH			
03/17/94	30400520	LOOP IV	9.68	9.68	
03/17/94	30400666	SPECIPAN COLLECT UNT	12.01	12.01	
03/17/94	30400699	ANGIOCATH 22G 1	7.87	7.87	
03/17/94	30401361	SET IV PUMP 01754-01	36.24	36.24	

BLUE CROSS OF VIRGINIA

INSURANCE BENEFITS ASSIGNED ▶

PATIENT
PLEASE PAY

DUE & PAYABLE UPON RECEIPT.

¤¤ REPRINT ¤¤ – 1S

THESE CHARGES DO NOT INCLUDE FEES FOR PROFESSIONAL SERVICES RENDERED. YOU WILL RECEIVE A SEPARATE BILL FROM THE PHYSICIAN.

PLEASE EXAMINE THIS STATEMENT CAREFULLY. THIS WILL BE YOUR ONLY ITEMIZED STATEMENT FOR THE ABOVE TRANSACTIONS. IF YOU HAVE ANY QUESTIONS CONCERNING THIS STATEMENT PLEASE CONTACT _____ ▶PATIENT ACCOUNTS Phone

Example of an itemized bill

bibliography at the back of the book, I've compiled a list of some of the most handy reference sites on the Internet.

Undoubtedly you'll run into some things (such as bundles and trays, which we'll discuss in the next chapter) that require a deeper level of understanding. If necessary, this

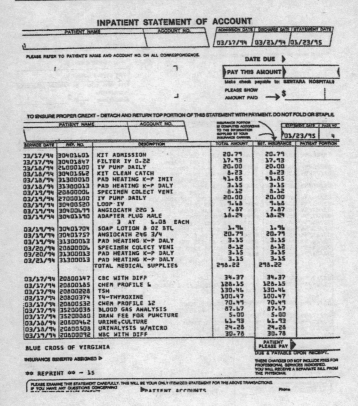

Example of an itemized bill

is where you may want to contact a medical billing advocate to work on your behalf.

INPATIENT STATEMENT OF ACCOUNT

PATIENT NAME		ACCOUNT NO.		ADMISSION DATE	DISCHARGE DATE	STATEMENT DATE
				03/17/94	03/21/94	01/23/95

PLEASE REFER TO PATIENTS NAME AND ACCOUNT NO. ON ALL CORRESPONDENCE.

DATE DUE ▶

PAY THIS AMOUNT

Make check payable to: SENTARA HOSPITALS

PLEASE SHOW
AMOUNT PAID ──▶ $

TO ENSURE PROPER CREDIT – DETACH AND RETURN TOP PORTION OF THIS STATEMENT WITH PAYMENT. DO NOT FOLD OR STAPLE.

PATIENT NAME		ACCOUNT NO.		INSURANCE PORTION IS COMPUTED ACCORDING TO THE INFORMATION SUPPLIED BY YOUR INSURANCE CARRIER.	STATEMENT DATE	PAGE NO.
					01/23/95	5

SERVICE DATE	REF. NO.	DESCRIPTION	TOTAL AMOUNT	EST. INSURANCE	PATIENT PORTION
03/19/94	20800165	CHEM PROFILE 6	128.15	128.15	
03/19/94	20800532	CHEM PROFILE 12	70.49	70.49	
03/20/94	20800147	CBC WITH DIFF	34.37	34.37	
		TOTAL LAB	906.61	906.61	
03/17/94	13000051	CHEST TWO VIEWS	80.00	80.00	
		TOTAL X-RAY	80.00	80.00	
03/17/94	35200001	AEROSOL EQUIP INSTAL	20.22	20.22	
03/17/94	35200024	HEATED NEBULZR SETUP	37.07	37.07	
03/17/94	35200027	OXYGEN MAXIMUM DAILY	155.79	155.79	
03/17/94	35200029	AEROSOL TRMT X 1	37.74	37.74	
		2 AT 18.87 EACH			
03/17/94	35200057	CANNULA SET UP	10.09	10.09	
03/17/94	35200059	PULM BASELINE EVAL	26.28	26.28	
03/18/94	35200027	OXYGEN MAXIMUM DAILY	155.79	155.79	
03/18/94	35200029	AEROSOL TRMT X 1	94.35	94.35	
		5 AT 18.87 EACH			
03/19/94	35200027	OXYGEN MAXIMUM DAILY	155.79	155.79	
03/19/94	35200027	AEROSOL TRMT X 1	18.87	18.87	
03/20/94	35200027	OXYGEN MAXIMUM DAILY	155.79	155.79	
03/21/94	35200027	OXYGEN MAXIMUM DAILY	155.79	155.79	
		TOTAL RESPIRATORY SERVICES	1023.57	1023.57	
03/17/94	35200045	PEAK FLOW PER TEST	71.47	71.47	
03/18/94	35200045	PEAK FLOW PER TEST	71.47	71.47	
03/19/94	35200045	PEAK FLOW PER TEST	71.47	71.47	
03/21/94	35200076	P.F.S.WITH PRE&POST	384.46	384.46	
		TOTAL PULMONARY FUNCTION	598.87	598.87	

BLUE CROSS OF VIRGINIA

INSURANCE BENEFITS ASSIGNED ▶

⇎ REPRINT ⇎ – 15

PATIENT PLEASE PAY ▶

DUE & PAYABLE UPON RECEIPT.

THESE CHARGES DO NOT INCLUDE FEES FOR PROFESSIONAL SERVICES RENDERED. YOU WILL RECEIVE A SEPARATE BILL FROM THE PHYSICIAN.

PLEASE EXAMINE THIS STATEMENT CAREFULLY. THIS WILL BE YOUR ONLY ITEMIZED STATEMENT FOR THE ABOVE TRANSACTIONS. IF YOU HAVE ANY QUESTIONS CONCERNING THIS STATEMENT PLEASE CONTACT ▶PATIENT ACCOUNTS Phone:

Example of an itemized bill

YOU MAKE THE CALL

Whether it's an abbreviation, code, or scribble, if you can't figure it out, pick up the telephone and call. Then ask. That's your first and best line of defense.

As best you can, locate the person or department re-

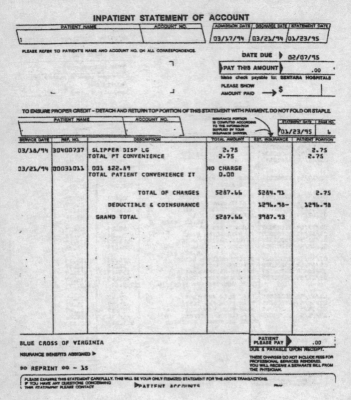

Example of an itemized bill

sponsible for the item and solicit their help. Get them on your side. Nurses are wonderful sources of information, and often they're more than willing to help. But they're busy people, so be respectful of their time. The same goes for doctors and other health care professionals.

Anytime you run into someone unwilling to help, politely move on to someone else.

And don't shy away from buying or borrowing reference books to look something up on your own.

But don't get going just yet.

At this point the stage is set, but you're still not quite ready to sing. You can't yet unlock many of the mysteries in your medical bill. The chapters that follow will show you the types of things for which you need to be on the lookout.

For now, keep in mind, it's steak you want, not brains and snails.

ACTION POINTS

❑ **If you don't know what something means, ask!** Don't let the foreign-sounding language of "medicalspeak" deter you. Be curious—it's your right and your responsibility.

❑ **Don't lose heart.** While the sight of your itemized medical bill may make you want to run for cover, don't. It's not as bad as it looks.

❑ **Order your medical records.** Send a brief, written request to the medical records department of your hospital. Check with them first to find out what fees (retrieval and copying) they will charge. Make sure their charges are within the legal limits of the state.

❑ **Get help.** Call. Read. Ask. Be polite, yet firm. But first, read the chapters ahead to uncover the types of mysteries buried within.

5

High Fever

HOW TO RECOGNIZE AND REDUCE EXCESSIVE CHARGES

Carolyn Albright needed a pacemaker, which was a problem wrapped inside a problem.

For six months she'd been fighting recurring heart palpitations and constant dizziness. Her health was declining daily. She couldn't wait any longer—she needed help, and she needed it now.

This worried Dr. Andrew Lusk.

The New England physician's patient was fifty-five years old. She and her husband were barely making ends meet on a very tight, fixed income, and they were already taking care of his ninety-two-year-old mother.

She had no health insurance.

Her heart was unstable.

And he had to tell her she needed a medical device that would cost her thousands of dollars.

Dr. Lusk gave Carolyn the bad news, then sat down with

her and her husband to discuss their financial options. There weren't many from which to choose. She had to have the pacemaker.

But Dr. Lusk promised he would do whatever he could to reduce costs on the couple's behalf. He tossed out some ideas.

As for the pacemaker itself, he said he could order an older, less expensive model for her as opposed to the latest, greatest state-of-the-art wondergadget. She really didn't need a Range Rover, he told her, when a Dodge Dakota would do her just fine.

She agreed.

Then, he believed, they could minimize the length of her hospital stay. At the time, most patients receiving pacemakers were being hospitalized for a minimum of forty-eight hours. He felt that if they timed it just right, and all went well, she could be out within one day.

That sounded great to her.

Furthermore, Dr. Lusk suggested that—again, if all went well—they could forgo monitoring her progress following the surgery, though normally that's done as standard procedure.

She had no problem with that.

The day of Carolyn Albright's surgery came and all went well: No complications, and she was released from the hospital twenty-three hours after she arrived. She had made it in and out in one day as hoped.

But her attempts at frugality had gone unrewarded, she realized later when she received her hospital bill.

The total came to $17,560.50.

A twenty-three-hour hospital stay. A flawless surgical procedure. An older model pacemaker. No nonessential tests. No follow-up monitoring.

And *still* it cost her more than $17,000.

Her heart may have been healthier, but it had never been heavier than the day she contacted me for help.

Where there's smoke, I've learned, there's usually fire, and Carolyn's case proved no different. What could possibly have caused her bill to be so high?

Upon closer inspection, I found that nearly $14,000 of the $17,560.50 she owed her hospital was attributed to the cost of the pacemaker itself.

I called the company that supplied the pacemaker, and they quoted me a list price of $8,550 for that particular model! They then went on to tell me that the hospital's discount price was only $6,700!

So Carolyn's hospital had marked up the cost of a $6,700 pacemaker an additional $7,034.30, charging her almost $14,000 for an older-model device.

I'd have hated to see what they charge for something newly on the market!

As Dr. Lusk later wrote to me, "We went far beyond what's generally offered to try to minimize the expense of Carolyn's hospitalization and procedure." Unfortunately, he said, he couldn't control what the hospital charges.

"We have all been very concerned about the markup on pacemakers," he said. "The hospital chooses to continue this practice. While it may not be out of line compared to other hospitals, I have often been bothered by the degree of markup that we have observed as well."

CAVEAT EMPTOR

Whatever happened to the time-honored medical principle of "first, do no harm"? Clearly, as in the case of Carolyn

Albright, that time has come and gone. From a financial point of view, at least, it's passé.

Thankfully for Carolyn, after we let her hospital know that *we* knew how little her overpriced pacemaker had actually cost them, they were more than willing to negotiate. They didn't want us creating an uproar and spreading the word to other patients. Within a matter of hours they literally cut the total amount she owed in half!

But for every Carolyn out there, there are tens of thousands of other patients who never even realize they're being had. They're routinely paying markups of 100 percent, sometimes even *1,000* percent or more, and they're none the wiser.

It's just not right.

If I had to choose one principle that the medical community honors above all today, "first, do no harm" would certainly *not* come to mind.

It would be *caveat emptor*—"let the buyer beware."

We're all concerned with the ballooning cost of health care in this country. Good care comes with a price tag, of course . . . but shouldn't that price tag have some basis in reality?

Apparently not.

Here's another clear example of the medical establishment's distorted vision. One hospital in Illinois routinely charged $4,000 for cataract surgery. This procedure is usually done today as an outpatient surgery. The patient comes in for morning surgery and is out by the afternoon.

Patients were always complaining about the high hospital costs tacked on to what was a relatively straightforward surgical procedure.

The ophthalmologists who attended these patients agreed. They decided to open up an independent ambulatory center to perform these outpatient surgeries for their patients in a more economic manner. Without the hospital's charges, the doctors believed they could keep their patients' costs down to around $925 per surgery.

The hospital wasn't amused. They brought out their big legal guns and lobbied hard against the group's petition for a certificate of need from the state. (Every new hospital must prove to the state that its services are needed in a given area. The awarding of a certificate of need is the state's way of legally licensing a facility to do business.)

Lo and behold, in the midst of all the legal wrangling, the hospital that had been steadfastly charging $4,000 for cataract surgery decided it could still make a profit charging just $1,900!

Pacemakers and cataract surgeries are just a couple of big-ticket items made bigger by inflated prices. They are glaring violations of ethical business conduct.

But remember, the devil still lurks in the details.

Hospitals routinely inflate the smaller items too—and these violations, one could argue, are even more insidious because they're harder to bring to light.

For example, I found one hospital charging $444.78 for a 10-milligram vial of the neuromuscular blocking drug Norcuron. Overpriced? All I know is this: I found another hospital charging $17.90 for the very same 10-milligram vial.

Four hundred and forty-four dollars versus seventeen. You make the call.

ADMINISTRATION FEES (PAYING TO GET IN)

Believe it or not, some hospitals begin overcharging their patients before they even admit them.

How can that be?

Some charge what they call an "admission" or "administration" fee. This fee ostensibly covers the cost for the forms a patient signs prior to admission.

These are the forms on which they record your insurance information and your life history and your spouse's life history and your nephew's place of employment—all so they'll know where to go to collect on your bill should you default. I'm being a bit facetious, of course . . . but this is also where they have you unknowingly sign away all your earthly rights!

Think I've become a bit jaded?

Maybe so, but I've seen some of these "administration" fees go as high as $170! What, are they etching these forms onto gold tablets? Are they charging by the letter?

Sometimes this fee will include the initial assessment done by the nurse once you arrive at your room (at which point she checks what medications you're taking, who they'll need to contact in the case of an emergency, etc.). But oftentimes it doesn't even cover that.

RENT-TO-OWN EQUIPMENT

If hospitals allowed patients to take home every piece of equipment for which they were charged during their hospital stay, each patient would probably need to rent a U-Haul truck to get it all home.

Why would that be?

I'll let Rick Wade, spokesman for the American Hospital Association, tell you himself. "Under the crazy system that we have," he says, "all of the costs of everything that keeps a hospital able to serve twenty-four hours a day is hidden behind items that you can measure on a bill."

Let's unpack the meaning in that statement.

For one thing, it means you end up paying $18.50 for the same stick of deodorant that you can buy from your local drugstore for $2.50. (And you're lucky if you even use it two or three times.)

It also means you end up paying $20 for a $4 shoehorn.

And you might be paying up to $130 *per day* for the use of a piece of equipment like a patient-controlled analgesia (PCA). (That's the pump device that allows a patient to self-administer more morphine at the push of a button.) Or $60 per day for the use of another sophisticated piece of equipment commonly called an electric blanket.

It can even mean you get charged rental fees on equipment far above and beyond what you would have paid had you actually *bought* the equipment.

Outpatient equipment is notorious in this regard. For example, if when you leave the hospital your doctor has recommended you use a wheelchair, walker, or cane, you will probably pay a home health agency a monthly rental fee for the equipment—say, $8.50 per month for a cane. After six months or so, though, it's not uncommon for your rental fees to have surpassed the cost of *buying* the cane (maybe $40). But the home health agency keeps charging, and you keep paying, and the equipment remains the agency's property!

Medicare and other forms of insurance won't pay a dime beyond the actual cost of the equipment, so why should anyone else have to?

Go figure.

But you can also get charged rental fees for equipment

that's just occupying space during your stay in your hospital or operating room.

For instance, I've seen patients charged $5.40 apiece for the little plastic covers put over the lights' handles in the operating room, which probably cost the hospital pennies.

Speaking of the OR, surgical tools typically come prepackaged into trays. Patients are almost always charged for the full cost of the tray. Even though the surgeon might use only two or three of the tools during the operation, the hospital passes on the cost of every tool every time. We'll discuss this practice in more detail later when we look at the issue of hidden charges.

Then there's the man who discovered that his wife was charged $785 for an intern training video taken in the OR during her gallstone surgery. Talk about being overcharged—he never even got a copy of the video! (Unfortunately, video charges aren't all that uncommon.)

THE TROUBLING SIGNS OF DRUG ABUSE

Financial personnel within hospitals have told me that the money hospitals make by marking up the price of drugs alone covers *one-third to one-half* of the hospital's total overhead.

That's terrifying to me.

To see just how much money hospitals are making off of medications, compare the price of a single pill on your bill to the cost of that same pill bought over-the-counter at your local drugstore.

If drug companies are making healthy profits by selling aspirin at those over-the-counter prices, think of how much profit is being made by hospitals charging ten and twenty times more!

Compare, for instance, the cost of one throat lozenge. A hospital can buy one Cepacol throat lozenge wholesale for 4.5 cents. But they might turn around and bill you $2.25 or more per lozenge.

The market value of a 5-milligram dose of the drug Reglan is around 45 cents. Hospitals routinely charge $4 or more. Even as I write this sentence, I can glance over at a client's bill and see where her hospital charged her $3 per single Tylenol tablet.

Do you know what's really sad? That kind of thing hardly even fazes me anymore! Such overblown charges are the rule, not the exception.

Hospitals make excuses for why they charge so much for their medications. They claim the high prices are necessary to cover their pharmacy department's cost of ordering, stocking, and dispensing the drugs.

I think Rick Wade's explanation is the one that hits the nail on the head. Hospitals are hiding *all* the costs they can behind those drugs.

And then some.

Here's further proof. One charge you may run into is called an "oral administration fee." What that means is they're charging you for the nurse to put your pills in that little white cup and hand them to you. That's an "oral administration fee."

Ironically, that's a service—just like any other nursing service—covered under your hospital room and board charge. It's services like those, they say, that make your room charge so high.

Think about that. You're paying for the nurse's service as part of your room and board. Then you're paying for it again as an "oral administration fee." Then you're paying $4 or $5 for the pill she gives you, which in reality only costs pennies.

That's not health care. That's insanity.

The excuse that hospitals give for charging so much for room and board is the same excuse they give for charging so much for medication, which is the same excuse they give for coming up with such ridiculous charges as "oral administration fees."

What they're doing is having their cake and eating it too.

And they're putting it on your tab and mine.

DOCTORING THE BILL

Sometimes the doctors themselves get into the action.

For instance, if a surgeon happens to perform three procedures during the course of one operation, the patient will sometimes be charged for three separate operations, each at full price.

Medicare and other forms of insurance don't allow this. Standard policies dictate that the surgeon charge full price for only one procedure, then *half* price for the other two.

Oftentimes this separate billing glides undetected below third-party payers' radar. But if you catch it, the difference in cost can be significant.

Routine office visits to your doctor can be trouble as well. Physicians are supposed to bill office visits to Medicare and other insurers according to the actual face time they spend with their patient. It's common, though, for doctors to charge an office visit of twenty minutes or more when they only spend five minutes in the room face-to-face with a patient.

THE WEAPONS WE FIGHT WITH

So now you have an idea of the many ways in which hospitals and doctors can inflate the prices of items both large and small right out of the stratosphere.

Unfortunately, no laws exist to prevent doctors and hospitals from doing this. They can keep sticking it to us any way they can as long as we let them.

The responsibility to keep our medical costs in check falls on our shoulders.

To defend ourselves, we should use whatever weapons we can, and the single most powerful weapon we have is information. We need not be afraid to call around, even to hospital suppliers, to get accurate pricing information.

Having good information in hand enables us to wield another powerful weapon—*leverage*. Our hospitals don't want people to know how much money they're making off each item, and we can use their fear of exposure to our advantage. More often than not, they would rather negotiate quietly than battle publicly.

ACTION POINTS

□ **Take the lead.** Don't expect the government or your insurance company or your HMO to deflate the inflated prices on your medical bill. There's no law preventing the exaggerated prices. The responsibility is yours alone.

□ **Compare prices.** You do it when you're buying a car. You do it when you're buying groceries. You should do it when you're buying medical care. Even if you failed to shop around before buying, comparing prices after the fact can still reap rewards. Knowledge is power.

□ **Especially for big-ticket items, call your hospital's purchasing department to find out from whom they're buying.** That way you can find out exactly what they're paying. You don't need to tell the purchasing agent that you're investigating the charges on your hospital bill. Let them know it's vital you get the information, but let them guess as to the reason why. (Maybe you need to purchase another one just like the one you've already bought?)

❏ **Call suppliers directly.** Ask them how much they charge. Do they offer discounts to hospitals? Bulk rates? What's their lowest price?

❏ **Leverage what you know.** Sit down with the financial director of your hospital and kindly yet firmly share the difference between their asking prices and the costs they actually paid. Remember, they'd rather negotiate and have you keep your information to yourself than risk others finding out. Even if they won't budge on some items, you'll still have added leverage in your favor when you discuss other problem areas with them, such as duplicate and hidden charges.

Here and elsewhere, always . . .

❏ **Be polite.** Remember, if you want honey, it does you no good at all to kick over the beehive.

6

Double Vision

HOW TO RECOGNIZE AND REMOVE DUPLICATE CHARGES

Some months ago, a news report on National Public Radio caught my attention.

"Recently, the Health and Human Services inspector general completed an investigation into fraudulent billing among hospitals," the reporter began.

I was all ears.

"The findings were shocking," she said. "Forty-six hundred of the nation's 5,000 hospitals—nearly all of them—were billing Medicare twice for the same service. The government has settled 2,000 of those cases so far and forced the hospitals to repay $45 million. The expected recovery, once all cases are settled, is about $120 million."

In that report, Kirk Nahra, general counsel for an organization called the National Health Care Anti-Fraud Association, pointed out a disturbing trend: "When you looked at fraud ten or fifteen years ago, what you tended to see was a focus on providers that were at the periphery of the profession. That is not true today. There are fraud investigations going on against the most respected health care providers in the country."

Forty-six hundred out of our 5,000 hospitals, to be exact . . . to the tune of $120 million!

Interestingly, the Justice Department is nailing these hospitals for violating something called the False Claims Act, a law first enacted during the Civil War to keep horse traders from selling the same horse to the government twice.

The more things change, the more they stay the same.

This news story gives us a little insight into the severity of the problem of double-billing among medical facilities in America.

One would hope, even expect, that if these providers are getting caught, they're cleaning up their acts. One would think that if the government is making these crooks pay so much money, the fraud they're perpetrating is screeching to a halt.

Much as we'd like to think so, it's not.

While medical providers are being more careful how they bill Medicare, they are still double-dipping left and right when it comes to billing patients and private insurers. I know because I see it being done every day.

BUNDLES OF FUN

The most common way providers—hospitals and medical laboratories, mainly—double-bill their patients is through a billing practice known as *unbundling*.

Simply put, unbundling occurs when hospitals and laboratories bill patients separately for tests or procedures that are performed—and are supposed to be billed—together (as a bundle).

A "Chem-7" is just such a bundle. A Chem-7 is a blood test commonly ordered by doctors to check a patient's blood for potassium, for glucose, and for five other substances. Once the blood sample is taken, all seven of these tests are done at one time—automatically, as a bundle—and are billed together.

If patients were billed for each of the seven tests individually, the total bill would be much higher. And the provider who billed them that way would be guilty of unbundling.

Buying a bundled test or procedure like a Chem-7 is not unlike buying a value meal at a fast-food restaurant. When you buy the sandwich, fries, and drink bundled together as Meal #1, the total cost is less than it would be if you bought each item separately. It's more convenient that way too, since the items sold together naturally go together.

(In case you're wondering who within the medical field decides what gets bundled and what doesn't, such decisions are made by physicians representing all specialties of medicine under the auspices of the American Medical Association. They also get input from third-party payers and government agencies.)

Here's some further insight into how unbundling works.

Medicare or a private insurance company may pay a doctor up to $210 for performing an upper gastrointestinal endoscopy, or a "GI" tube, as it's commonly called. (I say "may" because insurance rates vary from region to region and from company to company.) That same insurer may also pay the doctor up to $90 for a stomach biopsy.

But anytime the doctor performs an upper gastrointestinal endoscopy and a stomach biopsy during the same surgery—as is often the case—the doctor can only bill the patient's insurer for one charge under one code at a combined "value meal" rate of no more than, say, $240.

When a doctor bills for each procedure separately (for a total cost of $300 instead of the combined, allowable cost of $240), he is guilty of double-billing, of billing for an additional procedure when in reality that procedure was supposed to have been charged as part of another.

Congratulations. You and your insurer have just been unbundled. Unfortunately for you, more often than not, your insurer will *not* catch the error.

Sometimes such unbundling is done intentionally and sometimes it's not. *Intentional* unbundling occurs when the doctor attempts to manipulate the coding in order to maximize the amount he can get from the insurer. *Unintentional* unbundling occurs when a doctor innocently misinterprets which billing code should be used.

Whether it's done intentionally or not, the result of unbundling is always the same: Money that rightfully belongs to you and your insurer wrongfully goes into your doctor's pocket.

IN ONE NOSTRIL AND OUT THE OTHER

You're probably familiar with Charles Dickens's *A Tale of Two Cities*. But consider for a moment Bob Delaney and his tale of two sinuses. (Humor me, okay?)

A few years ago Bob moved from his native New Mexico to the scenic Shenandoah Valley of Virginia. After weathering the initial culture shock, Bob fell in love with his new surroundings—the mountains, the trees, the greenery, the changing seasons, and especially, the occasional snows.

However, though he was attracted to his new environment, Bob found himself allergic to it as well.

And so it was with an acute sinusitis that he went to see his doctor.

Bob needed surgery to help clean out his infected sinuses. Such a procedure is called a bilateral nasal endoscopy (in layman's terms, a two-nostril deep-sea plunge).

When Bob got a whiff of his bill, he was ready to head back West. He owed over $6,300 in surgeon's fees alone!

He asked me to investigate his bill, and I did.

I noticed immediately that his doctor had billed him $4,057 for one *bilateral* nasal endoscopy *and* billed him $1,203 for an additional *unilateral* nasal endoscopy.

Aha. Bob had been unbundled.

When I asked Bob's doctor why he had charged for two nasal endoscopies during the course of one surgical procedure, he explained that after having done the original bilateral endoscopy as planned, he decided to go back in and clean out the base of Bob's nasal cavity. And bill Bob for the extra effort, of course.

Insurers have a word they use for this kind of double-billing: *no*.

At least that's what they say whenever they can catch it. And that's exactly what we said to Bob's doctor when we caught it.

PACKAGED DELIVERIES

Any item that's "packaged" on your bill ought really to stir your curiosity. For instance, a new mother who delivered her baby via a cesarean section might notice a charge on her bill for something called a "C-Section Tray." That C-Section Tray would have consisted of surgical tools her obstetrician used during the baby's delivery. It might have included the following items packaged together:

C-SECTION TRAY CONTENTS

E.S. PENCIL, BUTTON W/HOLSTER

BLADE, #10 CS

YANKUER, HNDL. BULB TIP, NV

CONN.TUBE, 20X3/16"

LITE GLOVE

BAG, SUTURE

BAG, HEADER 23X35

BASIN, RING 6.5 LITER

WRAP, SPUNGUARD 54X72

PAD, MATERNITY

SYRINGE, IRR.60CC (D20127)

BOWL, SPONGE 64OZ BLUE (62002)

TRAY, MAYO 16X21

DRAPE, HALF 41X70

DRAPE, THREE QUARTER

SYRINGE, 30CC

WRAP, POLY WRAP

SYRINGE, EAR

NDL.COUNTER

TOWEL, BLUE CLOTH

TOWEL CLIP

CORD CLAMP

TRAY, 10X5X2

GOWN, XLG.SPECIAL

DRAPE, C-SECTION

TAPE, ETP INDICATOR

LAP SPONGE, 18X18

TABLE COVER, 70X11

MAYO COVER

CONTAINER, SPEC.40

The total charge for such a C-Section Tray might come to about $200. But if she looks closely at her itemized statement, she may realize that she also received separate charges for a "MATERNITY PAD" and a "CORD CLAMP" totaling an extra $42. These are extra charges, of course, because she was already charged for these items when she paid for the C-Section Tray.

Likewise, a person who had cataract surgery might receive a $400 charge for something called a "Mini-Cataract Pack" (shown below) and yet uncover an additional $70 in charges for the two crescent knives included in the pack.

MINI-CATARACT PACK

PHACO PAK	PROCEDURE TRAY
I-SPEAR	10CC SYRINGE
3MM ANG FULL HANDLE	5CC SYRINGE
OPHTHALMIC DRAPE	NEEDLE 18 X 1 1/2
BIPOLAR BRUSH	NEEDLE 25 X 1 1/2
IRRIGATING CYSTITOME	CSR WRAP
ANT CHAMBER CANNULA	PROCEDURE TRAY
10-0 BMN SUTURE	TB SYRINGE W/NEEDLE
RETRO NEEDLE	SURGEONS GLOVES 7½
4-0 SILK SUTURE	COTTON TIP APPLICATOR
CRESCENT KNIFE	DRAIN, EYE W/COLLECTION BAG
CRESCENT KNIFE	SUTURE
HAND BAGGIE	RUBBER BAND

This sort of duplicate billing happens much too often. In my experience, rarely is it done unintentionally.

If you see anything on your bill labeled a "tray," a "package," or a "pack," find out what's included in the package and check to make sure that none of those items are included on your bill as a separate charge.

As necessary as some of those items might be, you don't need to be paying twice for any of them! (As it is, you're already paying a lump sum for a pack of items most of which your doctor never used.)

GARBAGE IN, GARBAGE OUT

The most obvious (and often the most comical) examples of double-billing often are due to clerical errors—the product of data-entry workers who simply strike the wrong keys on their computers.

That's how, for instance, the Illinois man we heard about in the first chapter was billed a whopping $186,000 for 200 heart valves, when he was supposed to have been billed for only two.

Such gross errors are easy to spot on an itemized bill and, of course, easy to rectify. (You just point to them and ask, "What is *this*?")

Other examples might include being billed for 36 hours' use of oxygen in one 24-hour day. Or, as I saw on one newborn baby's bill, 150 gauze pads (6 boxes, 25 pads per box). While I wouldn't mind having a 36-hour day every now and again, I definitely wouldn't want to give birth to a baby large enough to have that much blood to lose!

TAKING PICTURES . . . FURTHER

One common (and less obvious) form of double-billing is done routinely by radiology departments all across the nation.

Anytime you have to have an X ray retaken, beware. No matter what the cause—no matter who's to blame—*anytime* you have to have an X ray retaken, you will probably be asked to pick up the tab for the additional shots.

Maybe it so happened that the film was bad. Or maybe the film didn't develop properly. Or maybe the radiology technician screwed up. Or maybe the radiologist took two or three views when the doctor only ordered one.

It doesn't matter.

Regardless of the cause, the effect is *you* get charged for *their* mistakes.

Likewise, if you have an electrocardiogram (EKG) taken, and for some reason your name is not affixed to the tape (as sometimes will happen), the EKG might need to be taken again. And again, you'll pay twice for the same test.

Remember, without an itemized statement you'll never notice these duplicated charges. On a summary bill, all such charges are lumped under a single category, such as "radiology." And for the most part, that lumped charge is what your insurer pays.

It isn't right, but it's common practice.

While we're on the subject of radiology, keep in mind, too, that if you have an X ray taken after normal business hours, you'll probably be charged twice for the reading of that one X ray: one for the emergency room physician reading it that night, another for the radiologist's "professional" reading the next day.

And that's not even to mention the fact that there are usually two bills for every X ray done during the day: In addition to the professional charge (what the radiologist charges to read your X ray), you usually pay a *technical* charge too (covering the "cost" of your use of their equipment!).

Too often I've seen people charged for both services, when in reality only one is rendered.

DOCTOR, DOCTOR, GIVE ME THE NEWS

I'd be a wealthy woman if only I had a dime for every time a frustrated client has come into my office and complained, "I've been billed by doctors I've never even heard of."

Do such complaints have any merit?

Let me just say this: Beware the friendly doctor who pops his head into your hospital room (while you're lying there half-conscious) to say hello.

That can be a costly greeting. Some doctors have been known to stop by a room, glance over a patient's chart, pause ever so studiously, then walk out, never to be seen again.

Until, mysteriously, their name shows up on a bill for "consultation"!

Sometimes it turns out that's the "doctor I've never heard of." I'd say that when a doctor bills you for a service that another doctor is already providing, that's a pretty clear-cut case of double-billing.

Other times, though, the "doctor never heard of" can play a more substantive role in a patient's care, and can double-bill them more substantively, too.

For instance, often a surgeon is assisted in surgery by

a fellow practitioner. Expect the assistant surgeon to send you a bill as well. But the fun doesn't stop there. Often this assistant surgeon will charge the same rate that the primary surgeon charged, even though standard Medicare and insurance guidelines dictate he only charge *20 percent* of the primary surgeon's charge.

Why do they do it? Think about it. How often will insurance companies actually catch this error? Not very. And how many people without insurance will even know this is an illegitimate charge? Not many.

I wish that someone could give me a good explanation why surgeons aren't required to notify patients ahead of time that an assistant will be attending the surgery—and required to tell the patient that they will be incurring an extra charge for the assistant's services!

Isn't that just plain common sense? Maybe so, but it's by no means common practice.

Last year, the University of Pennsylvania Hospital repaid Medicare $30 million in an out-of-court settlement. The hospital admitted no wrongdoing. But the accusation that had been leveled against them? The government claimed the hospital had been billing Medicare for the services of experienced physicians when the care was actually being delivered by less experienced residents-in-training.

Thirty million dollars is a lot to pay for no wrongdoing.

CAUGHT IN THE MIDDLE

Here's a doctoral-level puzzle of a different sort.

I go into the operating room for one procedure, but when

I awaken in the recovery room my doctor informs me he performed two additional procedures he felt were medically necessary to alleviate my pain.

That makes sense. I trust his judgment. He's the surgeon, right?

But the pain returns when my insurance company disputes my doctor's professional opinion and denies my claim for the additional procedures. They refuse to pay.

The doctor blames the insurer, the insurer blames the doctor, and I'm left holding the bill. I don't know who's right and who's wrong. I was lying on my back in la la land during the surgery and had absolutely no say whatsoever in the matter.

Yet *I'm* the one held responsible.

I am the one sent to the collection agency. *I* am the one with the ruined credit record. *I* am the one who now can't get a loan to buy a new home.

And I was the *only* one who was unconscious at the time the decision was made!

Gives a whole new meaning to the phrase "you snooze, you lose," doesn't it?

WHERE TO TURN FOR HELP

When we go on vacation and stay at a hotel, we may pay out $100 a night or more. What are we paying for? We're paying for the room, the bed, the shower, the soap. We're paying for the maids to change the bedsheets, to empty the trash, to scrub the sink, to replenish the towels.

We usually have no problem paying the daily room rate because we know that built into it are a host of services we need taken care of.

And so they are.

But such is definitely *not* the case when we stay overnight in a hospital. Remember, hospitals justify charging exorbitant room rates—$300 to $500 or more—by claiming the charge covers such services as housekeeping and nursing services in addition to room and board. Yet patients still get billed for some of these services. (Remember the "oral administration fee" where a patient pays for the nurse simply to hand him a pill? Remember the $60-per-day charge for the use of an electric blanket?)

So we end up allowing our local hospital to charge us a daily room rate higher than that of a posh hotel at an exotic beach locale, then we allow them to charge us a second time for many of the same services.

Whose fault is it, really?

If we're not taking full responsibility for our own medical finances, it's hard to point the finger of blame toward others.

Our hospitals and our insurance companies are taking advantage of us for reasons as scary as they are simple: First, they know they can; second, they've been doing it for years.

I know I repeat myself, but I feel I must. The first person to turn to for help is yourself. *You* need to get an itemized bill. *You* need to review each and every item on that bill. *You* need to question anything and everything you see but don't understand.

ACTION POINTS

❏ **Unwrap the bundles.** If someone tells you that a particular term on your bill refers to a bundled test or procedure, find out exactly what items are included in that bundle and check to make sure none of those items reappear elsewhere on your bill as a separate charge.

❏ **Disassemble the packages.** When you come across a "tray," a "package," or a "pack," you need to ensure that none of the items included in that package are also being charged separately.

❏ **Decline all extraneous photos.** When you come upon radiology charges, make sure the radiology department isn't charging you for some of their mistakes.

❏ **Unveil the mystery doctors.** When you get a bill from a "doctor you've never heard of," you need to find out who he was and what specific services he actually provided. How? Call him. Ask him. Make him show you some documentation. (As we'll learn shortly, if a service wasn't documented, it wasn't done.) Did the mystery doctor just pop his head in your room for a moment? Then challenge his charge. Did he serve as an assistant to your surgeon during surgery? Then make sure he isn't charging you any more than 20 percent of the fee you're paying your primary surgeon.

7

Internal Bleeding
HOW TO RECOGNIZE AND REVEAL HIDDEN CHARGES

We live in a euphemistic society. MMMMMMMMMM We temper our words, we select them carefully, we make them politically correct—so as not to offend anyone with our language. We're always coming up with new words and phrases to replace older ones that have taken on negative connotations.

For instance, those whom we once called handicapped we now call "physically challenged." Those whom we once called deaf we often call "hearing impaired." Some go so far as to call those whom we once called bald "follically-challenged." (I still say bald.)

Because men and women now perform many of the jobs once relegated to only one sex, stewardesses have given way to "flight attendants," firemen have turned into "firefighters," and waiters and waitresses have both become "wait staff."

Because we more fully recognize that everyone likes to feel their job has inherent value, secretaries are now "administrative assistants," retail sales clerks have become "associates," and janitors have evolved into "maintenance engineers."

Most of the time such creative wordsmithing is done with good intention, out of genuine respect for others. Sometimes, however, people play fast and loose with language just to suit their own needs—simply to make a buck.

And so it is we find used cars advertised as "previously owned," added salt packaged as "minerally enhanced," and pornography peddled as "adult entertainment."

POLITICALLY INCORRECT

As we've already seen, hospitals and other health care facilities employ a form of political correctness all their own. And, more times than not, in so doing they resemble the used-car dealer more than they do the office manager.

Often our health care providers choose to employ certain language solely to help them make bigger bucks. And they can be pretty darn creative in the ways they do it, too.

Think back to an example we discussed earlier. What patient in his or her right mind would willingly pay a nurse $5 just to hand over a pill—again and again and again? Would *you* be willing to pay a bill that read like this?

Date of Service	Description of Service	Total Charge
01/01	001 16310013 NURSE HANDED YOU A PILL	5.00
01/01	001 16310013 NURSE HANDED YOU A PILL	5.00
01/01	001 16310013 NURSE HANDED YOU A PILL	5.00
01/01	001 16310013 NURSE HANDED YOU A PILL	5.00
01/01	001 16310013 NURSE HANDED YOU A PILL	5.00
01/01	001 16310013 NURSE HANDED YOU A PILL	5.00
01/01	001 16310013 NURSE HANDED YOU A PILL	5.00
01/01	001 16310013 NURSE HANDED YOU A PILL	5.00
01/01	001 16310013 NURSE HANDED YOU A PILL	5.00
01/01	001 16310013 NURSE HANDED YOU A PILL	5.00
01/01	001 16310013 NURSE HANDED YOU A PILL	5.00
01/01	001 16310013 NURSE HANDED YOU A PILL	5.00

I wouldn't pay this bill. And I doubt seriously if you would either.

Yet I know countless patients—and countless insurance companies too—who will pay a bill that reads like this, without ever blinking an eye:

Date of Service	Description of Service	Total Charge
01/01	001 16310013	
	ORAL ADMIN FEE	5.00
01/01	001 16310013	
	ORAL ADMIN FEE	5.00
01/01	001 16310013	
	ORAL ADMIN FEE	5.00
01/01	001 16310013	
	ORAL ADMIN FEE	5.00
01/01	001 16310013	
	ORAL ADMIN FEE	5.00
01/01	001 16310013	
	ORAL ADMIN FEE	5.00
01/01	001 16310013	
	PO ADMIN FEE	5.00
01/01	001 16310013	
	PO ADMIN FEE	5.00
01/01	001 16310013	
	PO ADMIN FEE	5.00
01/01	001 16310013	
	PO ADMIN FEE	5.00
01/01	001 16310013	
	PO ADMIN FEE	5.00
01/01	001 16310013	
	PO ADMIN FEE	5.00

What's the difference between the two bills? Apart from the creative codespeak used on the second bill, of course, these bills are one and the same.

It's all in a name.

An "oral administration fee," if you recall, is the hospital's "politically correct" way of saying that the patient is being charged for a nurse to hand him a pill. And the abbreviation "PO" in this case means "by mouth"—so "PO ADMIN FEE" is just one more way of saying the very same thing.

(Remember, too, on top of this charge the patient will also be billed a separate charge for the pill itself and will also be billed a room rate that supposedly includes the nurses' services.)

DISPOSABLE MUCOUS RECOVERY SYSTEMS (AND OTHER SNOTTY TERMS)

Though I haven't seen the actual documentation, I recently came across mention of one hospital billing patients for use of something they called "disposable mucous recovery systems."

Can you guess what a "disposable mucous recovery system" is? It's actually a common household product. Most of us recognize it by a popular brand name: Kleenex.

That's right: A "mucous recovery system" is a box of tissues.

(If I had been that hospital, I think I would have called it a "disposable mucous *defense* system." Who wants to "recover" snot? Most of us are content just to be protected from it!)

But it's their chicanery, not mine.

Laugh if you want, but if memory serves, the difference in price between an ordinary box of facial tissues and a "disposable mucous recovery system" was nothing to sneeze at.

Here are just a few other scientific-sounding terms—and the very ordinary items that may be hidden behind them:

The Term	Is Probably Hiding . . .
"Thermal Therapy"	A plastic bag filled with ice cubes
"Cotton Professional"	A Q-tip
"Gauze Collection Bag"	A plastic trash bag
"Brace"	An elastic bandage
"Cough Support Device"	A teddy bear

PAYING TO EXHALE

I remember hearing a hard-hitting public service announcement from the American Lung Association that said, "When you can't breathe, nothing else matters but your next breath."

Unfortunately, when you can't breathe—*and you're lying in a hospital bed*—that next breath might cost you a small fortune.

Hey, whatever it takes, many would say.

But just what *does* it take?

Let's examine. Obviously, if you're in a hospital and you need oxygen, you'll be asked to cover the cost of the tube that brings the oxygen into your nose. (Few of us would prefer to cut costs by trying to recycle the tube that had been in the nose of the patient before us.)

You'll probably also be charged an "oxygen setup" fee that covers the cost of the complicated procedure in which the nurse or respiratory therapist reaches over to the wall behind you and switches the oxygen valve from the "off" position over to the "on" position.

And you'll need to pay for the oxygen itself. Oxygen may be precious, but it's also plenteous, and therefore quite affordable.

Except, that is, when your doctor prescribes it for you "as needed." The phrase "as needed," I believe, is hospital codespeak for "*cha-ching!*"

Why? Because when a doctor prescribes oxygen as needed, hospitals reserve the right to charge the patient every eight hours for oxygen, whether the oxygen is actually used or not. We've had hospitals tell us that as long as the oxygen valve is on and *ready* for use, they retain the right to charge as if it were being used.

So even if a patient never actually uses oxygen, it may still have been prescribed "as needed," and an oxygen charge (or, more accurately, oxygen *charges*) may be hiding somewhere on the patient's bill.

NEEDLEPOINT: ANOTHER WAY HOSPITALS STICK IT TO US

Not all billing viruses are airborne diseases. Some go straight into the bloodstream.

Let's revisit a basic hospital truth: The cost of nursing is included in a patient's daily room rate. Not only is that basic truth commonly violated with "oral administration fees" and "oxygen setup" fees, but hospitals tend to tack on an additional fee every time a nurse brings a needle into a patient's room.

Anytime a doctor, nurse, or phlebotomist adds medication to your IV or sticks a needle into your behind, you'll be stuck with a fee for the effort *above and beyond* the price of the medication being injected.

If your itemized bill contains any of the following charges, you've been stuck by a needle-related charge—a charge that hospitals generally keep buried beneath the skin of common knowledge:

- TOP IV ADM FEE
- INJ ADM FEE
- IM ADM FEE
- BLOOD COLLECTION
- VENIPUNCTURE

SPECIAL DELIVERIES

Once a patient's blood is drawn, it often has to be transported to an outside laboratory for analysis. Naturally, the patient covers the cost for that transportation. On a bill, such a charge might show up as a "COLLECTION/HANDLING FEE" or a "LAB HANDLING FEE."

But what's *not* so obvious is that these same fees are charged to the patient even when the lab work is done *internally*, meaning the patient is charged extra just to have a technician carry the tubes down the hall to the hospital lab.

Hospitals charge anywhere from $10 to $20 per carry for this service. (Unless, that is, your physician wants the results of the testing to come back quickly. In that case—which might show up as a "STAT" fee on your bill—you could pay $30 or more, even if your doctor doesn't actually see the results until he returns the next morning.)

CLEARING THE AIR

Smoke and mirrors are in no short supply on most major medical bills. Whether it be a bogus service, such as an "oral administration fee" or an "oxygen setup fee" or a "laboratory handling fee," or whether it be an overwhelming price for an underwhelming item, such as a glorified aspirin or cotton swab, some undesirable charge is tucked away on most every itemized bill.

And that's not even including the frighteningly large "MISCELLANEOUS" charge that occasionally rears its ugly head on many patients' summary bills. Paying that charge without investigating it is like going to the grocery store and handing the check-out clerk (excuse me, "associate") a blank check for "WHATEVER"!

How do you fight against this type of billing abuse? Once again, knowledge is power. You need to identify these charges and uncover their hidden meanings. You do that by asking.

But don't expect that just because you know what a lot of those crazy charges are, your hospital will rescind them. On the contrary, they'll do their best to justify them. Depending on the charge, for them to do otherwise might be tantamount to admitting fraud.

But this knowledge can still be of great importance to you. If you are challenging a hospital in some of the other areas we've mentioned in other chapters, this knowledge will add fuel to your collective fire. Even if they refuse to concede or lower some of these hidden charges, you've still built a stronger case for yourself in your overall bill negotiation.

ACTION POINTS

❏ **Overturn all the scientific-sounding rocks.** Remember our commonsense rule from chapter 4: If you don't know what something means, ask. Some ridiculous charges can be hiding behind innocuous-sounding descriptions, and it's up to you to uncover the hidden meanings. Otherwise, items like "oral administration fees" and "cough support devices" could pile up on you.

❏ **Make sure you aren't paying a price for the constant use of an item that was only prescribed "as needed."** Remember, an oxygen "as needed" order can be detrimental to your financial health—even if you never actually used any oxygen. Check also for related charges incurred by any therapist or lab worker.

❏ **Don't get "stuck" paying for services that you've already paid for.** Venipuncture charges and "oral administration fees" are prime examples. You do not need to pay for nursing services that should be covered under the umbrella charge of your room rate.

❏ **Transport fees.** If you've paid $20 or $30 or more just for someone to carry your test tubes down the hall, then your bloodwork wasn't the only thing that got taken! Make sure your lab work was actually transported somewhere before you agree to pay any type of transport fee.

8

Memory Loss
How to Recognize and Reject Undocumented Charges

One of the highest hurdles many hospitals must over-come along the track toward more accurate billing is a particularly sticky issue.

I mean that literally.

Attached to most medical supplies, you may have no-ticed, are little yellow stickers that contain coded identifi-cation and cost information.

Here's what such a sticker looks like:

```
46564
IRRIG NS 1000ML
2F7124
```

Nurses are supposed to remove these stickers at a pa-tient's bedside as supplies are used and then affix them immediately to a computer billing card (from which the information will eventually be transferred directly to the patient's account).

That's the way the sticker system is *supposed* to work, anyway.

In practice, sometimes these stickers make it to the billing card and sometimes they don't. Sometimes they get stuck on billing cards belonging to other patients. Sometimes they get stuck on the side of the patient's bed. Sometimes they get stuck on the wall (as I couldn't help but notice during my mother's illness, which you'll learn more about in the next chapter).

Often nurses temporarily plaster the stickers onto the fronts of their own uniforms while they're in the process of performing a service for a patient. The problem is, many times they walk out of the patient's room with those stickers still stuck to their uniforms!

What do the nurses do then?

Well, sometimes, if they catch their mistake in time, they return to the right patient's room and put the right sticker on the right billing card. At other times they might inadvertently stick them on the billing card of the next patient they see (along with that patient's stickers, which by that time have also been added to the front of the nurse's uniform). Sometimes nurses will try to track down the right patient but fail. Other times they may give up and toss the sticker in the nearest trash can.

Sound sloppy? It is.

Just walk into the cafeteria of any hospital that uses the sticker system, and I guarantee you'll see nurses with billing stickers stuck all over their uniforms. But in most hospitals, that's the system that's used.

Do we blame the nurses? I don't. They can hardly afford to pause long enough to put the stickers where they're supposed to go. Most nurses I know are usually running from one crisis to the next, meeting one need after another, doing the best they can. Their primary area of concern is patient *care*, not patient billing. Transferring stickers from supplies to billing cards is seldom the highest priority on a nurse's task list. Nor should it be.

Fortunately, some hospital systems are seeking to remedy this sad situation by going completely paperless. Everything from vital signs to syringe costs are electronically (and immediately) entered into a bedside computer, which is networked to a mainframe system.

"It saves time in transcription and it decreases the possibility of human error," said one executive in a hospital system pioneering the technology. But," he added, "we're just scratching the surface. We have a long ways to go, but someone has to scratch the surface."

Please keep scratching, sir. You may have a long way to go, but at least you're headed in the right direction.

IF IT ISN'T DOCUMENTED

Just how important are misplaced stickers to the cost of your care? Very. In the world of medical billing there is one universal rule recognized and honored by everyone who matters: *If it wasn't documented, it wasn't done.*

What does that mean, practically speaking?

It means that no matter what your doctor orders, whether it be a test, a procedure, a treatment, a supply, or a solution, or if an army of nurses gave it to you ten times a day for forty days and nights . . . anytime it wasn't documented as having been done, then as far as medical billing goes, it wasn't.

Consider that the next time you see a nurse walking down the hospital hallway with stickers hanging all over her uniform. What you are looking at are supplies that were never used!

But wait a minute. That isn't fair to the hospital, is it? If we used something, we ought to pay for it, right? That's only fair.

Of course it is.

But keep in mind the flip side of that fairness . . . when that same nurse sticks a couple of those stickers on *your* billing card when in reality they should have gone to the patient beside you!

That's just the way the sticky ball of supply charges bounces.

As for undocumented *services*, the issue isn't about what sticker goes where, but about which order was carried out and which wasn't. Were you given two Tylenol tablets every four hours (twelve total) per day as your doctor ordered, or were you only given eight? Was the dressing on that wound changed as often as he prescribed, or only half as often? Wouldn't you like to know, since you may be paying for the service regardless of whether the order was actually carried out or not?

How can a nurse remember a month or two later which orders were followed and which fell through the cracks? If she didn't write the service down as she performed it, she couldn't remember. That's why . . . *if it wasn't documented, it wasn't done*. If it's not written on your chart, you don't have to pay for it.

CHARTING YOUR COURSE

How on earth can you keep track of the services you paid for versus the actual services you received? It takes a bit of detective work, but almost always the time and effort are well spent.

The following chart is a simple tool I've developed to help people do just that. I call it a Hospital Log. This little chart is the heart and soul of medical bill error correction.

The log may look a bit scary, but actually it's as simple as one, two, three. Get out your medical records, then follow these three steps:

1) Go through your "Physician's Orders" sheet and transfer every order listed to the "DOCTOR'S ORDERS" column on the Hospital Log. List only one order per row, noting the date and time of each order in the adjoining columns.

2) Go through your "Nursing Notes," "Nursing Medication Sheet," "Laboratory Report," "X-ray Report," and "Therapy Notes" sheets and transfer every treatment, medication, and service listed on them to the "NURSE/LAB ORDERS" column on the Hospital Log. Go through the sheets one at a time, logging as you go each service rendered next to the specific doctor's order it fulfilled. Record the time and any pertinent notes beside each one in the appropriate columns.

3) Check the Hospital Log for discrepancies. Place a check mark in the "NOTES" column at the end of each row that has both a "DOCTOR'S ORDER" and a "NURSE/LAB/THERAPY NOTE" which documents that the order was carried out.

HOSPITAL LOG

Page 1 of 3 Pages

Patient: _____   Hospital: _____   Case Number: _____   Policy Yr: _____

Date	Time	DOCTOR'S Orders	NURSE/LAB Orders	Time	Notes
5/5/95	1315	INITIATED STANDARD ADMISSION ORDERS (same as NBC)	RECEIVED NEWBORN & INITIALIZED NEWBORN PLAN CARE (NBC same as SAO)	1315	
	1550	X-RAY PA & LATERAL CBC WITH DIFF BLOOD CULTURE			
			X-RAY PA & LAT-DONE	1600	
			CBC WITH DIFF - DONE	1630	
			BLOOD CULTURE - DONE		
			TRIPLE DYE (W/ NBC) - DONE	1730	
	1950	LAB: (1) URINE FOR GROUP B STREP (2) REPEAT CBC W/ DIFF IN AM (3) AMPICILLIN/ 175MG/ IM/ q12° (4) GENTAMYCIN/ 8MG/ IM/ q12°	CBC W/ DIFF RESULTS - WBC=50.6	1900	
			GENTAMYCIN/ 8MG /IM-DONE	2030	
			AMPICILLIN/ 175MG/ IM-DONE		

Example of Hospital Log

HOSPITAL LOG

Patient: _____ Hospital: _____ Case Number: _____ Page 2 of 3 Pages Policy Yr. ___

Date	Time	DOCTOR'S Orders	NURSE/LAB Orders	Time	Notes
5/6/95			GENTAMYCIN/ 8MG/ IM -DONE	1030	
	1035	REPEAT CBC W/ MANUAL DIFF	AMPICILLIN/ 175MG/ IM - DONE		
			LAB RESULTS - (1) URINE NEGATIVE (2) WBC = 37.0		
			GENTAMYCIN/ 8MG/ IM -DONE	2200	
			AMPICILLIN/ 175MG/ IM - DONE		
5/7/95			GENTAMYCIN/ 8MG/ IM -DONE	0845	
			AMPICILLIN/ 175MG/ IM - DONE		
			GENTAMYCIN/ 8MG/ IM -DONE	2030	
			AMPICILLIN/ 175MG/ IM - DONE		

Example of Hospital Log

HOSPITAL LOG

Page 3 of 3 Pages

Patient: _____ Hospital: _____ Case Number: _____ Policy Yr: _____

Date	Time	DOCTOR'S Orders	NURSE/LAB Orders	Time	Notes
5/8/95	0730	(1) PEAK & TROUGH GENTAMYCIN W/ LEVELS	LAB DREW - BLOOD	0814	
		(2) TYPE & COOMB ON CORD BLOOD	PEAK & TROUGH TYPE B+/ COOMBS NEGATIVE		
		(3) BILIRUBIN	BILIRUBIN		
		(4) CBC W/ DIFF	CBC W/ DIFF		
			GENTAMYCIN/ 8MG/ IM - DONE	0845	
			AMPICILLIN/ 175MG/ IM - DONE		
	1050	DISCHARGE HOME	DISCHARGED - HOME	1230	

Example of Hospital Log

A row that lacks either a doctor's order or a nurse's note is more than likely in error, because if an order wasn't documented, remember, it wasn't done. And likewise, any treatment that was given, but hadn't been ordered, wasn't done either. *You don't have to pay for services that weren't ordered.*

After you've finished logging your orders and notes, make a list of all the unchecked orders and services. Then pull out your itemized bill. Were you charged for these? If so, you shouldn't have been.

Make a list of these billing mistakes.

Now you'll want to take this list to your hospital billing office and ask them to either provide documentation for the orders/services or to remove the charges from your bill.

Easy enough? Just remember, as you go through your medical records, if you can't figure out what a word, phrase, code, or abbreviation means, find out. Call and ask someone directly, or look it up in an appropriate medical reference book.

HOUSTON, WE HAVE SOME PROBLEMS

The Hospital Log is a helpful tool that allows you to systematically list all of the items and services your hospital charged you for. I recommend you use it from the beginning of your medical billing investigation, but you can also find effective use for it at the end your investigation—for the purpose of review.

The following is a list of frequently found errors you should watch out for as you're filling out your Hospital Log, some of which we've already discussed, and some of which we haven't:

✓ Check to make sure no bundled items were billed separately from the prepared bundle, kit, pack, or tray in which they've already been included.

✓ Check to make sure you didn't get charged twice for lab or radiology tests that had to be repeated through no fault of your own.

✓ Unless you specifically requested a private room, you don't have to pay for one if that's where the hospital opted to place you. Check your room rate.

✓ Check to see if any items charged during your hospital stay had already been charged on your emergency room bill.

✓ Check to make sure no charges were billed before or after the time or date you were actually admitted. (I know it sounds crazy, but it happens much too often.)

✓ Check to make sure you weren't charged for too many gloves, too many coats, too many drapes, too many sutures, too many staples, too many *whatever*, during surgery. (If necessary, call or write your doctor and ask how many of the items in question were actually needed.)

When you're reviewing a bill from your doctor, you should also check for these specific problem areas:

✓ Check to make sure your doctor hasn't charged you for a hospital visit on the same day you had surgery. This "visit" should be included in the *surgical procedure fee*.

✓ Also check to make sure your doctor didn't charge you for your first visit back to his office following a surgery. That too is covered under the surgical procedure fee.

✓ Check to make sure you haven't been charged for a thirty- or forty-minute visit when you were only in the doctor's physical presence for ten. (This may be designated by a code, in which case you'll need to check with your doctor or nurse.)

✓ Check to make sure you don't already have a credit balance on your account. (If you do, you might even be so bold as to request interest for the time period during which your doctor's office had use of your money.)

✓ Check, too, for items and services already being billed from other offices: X rays, lab work, therapy, etc.

ACTION POINTS

❏ **Don't get tagged with someone else's stickers.**
While you're still in the hospital, if you can, have
someone keep a watchful eye out for those little
yellow stickers. Have them make sure your nurse
doesn't mistakenly give you a little yellow sticker
that happens to belong to another patient.

❏ **Create a Hospital Log.** Balance whatever has
been ordered by your doctor against everything
that actually was done.

❏ **If it wasn't documented, don't pay for it.** You
don't have to pay for any item, service, or procedure that's not clearly documented as having been
given or done in your medical records.

❏ **If it wasn't ordered, don't pay for it.** On the
other hand, no matter what a nurse, therapist,
technician, or anyone else has documented as
having been done for you, if your doctor never ordered it, you are not responsible for paying for it.
That goes for services, procedures, and supplies.

❏ **Balance your Hospital Log against your hospital
bill.** Were you charged for services ordered but never
performed? Were services performed that were never
ordered? Check your hospital bill to see if you were
charged for any of these possible errors.

❏ **Have your hospital billing department reconcile the differences.** Make them either provide
the documentation you've found lacking or remove
the charge. Remember, it's as simple as one, two,
three. Don't expect them to put up much of a fight
when you present them with cold hard facts!

9

The Big Picture
HOW HEALTH INSURANCE
WORKS TODAY

Last Thanksgiving I was exhausted, and so was every-one else in my family.

Business, which had long before become a family af-fair, was booming. We were being stretched this way and that, putting out one fire only to start another. And in the middle of the boom, just two weeks before the holiday, my eldest daughter, Candi, got married.

It was a beautiful wedding, but pulling it off took a lot out of us all (weddings will do that). On Thanksgiving Day, while Candi and her new husband were still in hon-eymoon mode, the rest of us were in recuperation mode!

We were enjoying a brief break between the hustle and bustle of wedding planning and the hustle and bustle of holiday shopping. All of us, that is, except my mother, who had come down with a bad cough. We suspected she'd caught bronchitis.

The day after Thanksgiving, Dad took Mom to the doctor. Her doctor suspected she might have pneumonia, not bronchitis, and he admitted her into the hospital. Tests there revealed that Mom had neither bronchitis nor pneumonia. She had something much worse: a tumor in the top part of one of her lungs. (Mom had been a smoker for over forty-five years.) Since the tumor was too deep to tell whether it was cancerous or not, her doctors elected to do surgery and take that part of her lung out. They removed what they could, but as it turned out, it was too little too late.

My mother was dead by Christmas. We were devastated.

Thankfully, Mom had medical insurance through a health maintenance organization. Under the terms of her membership, in the event of her hospitalization she was to pay a flat deductible of $300, and the HMO was to pay everything else.

Yet on the morning of his wife's funeral, as if he didn't have enough on his mind already, my father received a bill from the hospital for $10,000! He was shaken.

I was livid.

Two words were prominently plastered at the top of the statement: "NOW DUE." Another word, I noticed, was slipped in rather subtly at the bottom: "ESTIMATED." I tore the "bill" up and threw it in the garbage can before we left for the funeral home. "Don't even think about it," I told my dad. "Let's just go to the funeral."

A month later, Dad received a second statement. This time I called the hospital up on his behalf and told them, "My dad is seventy-one years old, he has a diseased heart, and you had better not send him any more bills until her insurance pays!"

He didn't get any more bills.

But four months after my mother's death, Dad did get

a statement from Mom's HMO. It was to notify him that they were covering all but $472 of her medical bills, in addition to her $300 deductible.

Four hundred and seventy-two dollars was not a huge sum in comparison to the total charge of $80,000 owed after all was said and done, but it wasn't chump change, either. The HMO was supposed to have covered *everything* beyond the deductible. I called the HMO and asked them just what it was they were refusing to cover.

Sixty-two dollars of the uncovered charge, it turned out, had been for a "blood pressure cup." Why the HMO chose not to cover that charge was beyond me, but since the hospital was under contract with the HMO to write off any necessary charges it didn't cover, the HMO saw to it that they did. The blood pressure cup was deemed necessary to my mother's care.

And the remaining $410? It turned out that money was for nicotine patches that my mother's doctor had prescribed for her to help her get through surgery without having to light up a cigarette. Her doctor had deemed them medically necessary in light of her condition.

But the HMO said no. The patches were items of *convenience*, they felt, and they wouldn't pay for them.

First things first.

Mom had been prescribed fifteen nicotine patches. The hospital had charged her *over $400* for fifteen nicotine patches. In other words, they had charged her almost $30 per patch . . . $30 for the very same patch you can buy at Wal-Mart for a little over a buck!

Before I even asked the HMO to pay for the patches, I called the hospital to complain about the price. Actually, I didn't just complain, I hit them where it could potentially hurt them the most: I threatened to go public with their price gouging.

"I think the news team down at Channel 7 might be interested in how much you're charging your patients for these little patches," I told them. Evidently they thought so too.

Dad was never billed for anything by anybody ever again.

Now allow me to let you in on a little secret.

I wasn't quite as good as I just made myself sound. Even though I work with hospital billing errors every day, and even though I've been fixing medical bills for years, when push came to shove in the case of my own mother's care, I still let the hospital and the HMO push me around.

How?

I was slow to react. Already grieving and not wishing to stir up even more unpleasantness, I put off making the calls I needed to. As a result, my father suffered from concerns he needn't have had in the first place.

Yes, in the end I did get the erroneous bill taken care of. But if I had it to do over again, I would have taken firmer control of the situation earlier. I wouldn't have waited days to rectify what could have been fixed in minutes.

I share this with you simply as an encouragement.

I know it can be tough. I've been there. Medical bills never come at a good time. They always hit you when you're down, when you're standing in the depths of the lowest valley with mountains of grief and pain rising high all around you, blotting out the light of the sun. Hope—and strength—can both seem so very far away.

But it's there in the valley that we must make our stand.

Hope *can* come again in the morning, but to be there to greet it, we have to stand firm through the night.

Standing firm is what this book is all about. These are battles we shouldn't have to fight; they're not of our own choosing, to be sure. But fight them we must.

My experience with my mother's illness helps illustrate, in a very small way, the bind in which patients and family members often find themselves, caught between the rock of hospitals and the hard place of insurers.

Up until this point, we've concentrated on the hospital side of medical bill survival. Now it's time we turned our attention to the other head of the medical billing beast: health insurance.

Because as bad as your hospital and doctors can hurt you financially, your insurance carrier can hurt you worse—especially when they don't cover bills you thought they should.

Before we even get into the specific problems patients generally will have to face when dealing with their insurers, we would do well to step back and remind ourselves of the overall insurance picture. It has changed a lot over recent years, and the pace of change isn't slowing anytime soon.

What are the different types of health insurance currently in vogue, and how does coverage differ between them? Let's take a quick look.

FEE-FOR-SERVICE COVERAGE

Most of us who have health insurance are covered one of two ways: either through a traditional *fee-for-service* plan or through a *managed care* plan.

A fee-for-service plan is one in which your insurance company pays your medical provider (your doctor or your hospital) a fee for each service rendered to anyone covered under your policy. You get to choose whatever doctor or hospital you want, and then either you or that provider submits each claim to the insurance company for reimbursement.

Any service rendered that's not listed in the benefits summary of your insurance policy will not be reimbursed. Any service that is listed will be reimbursed, though usually not at 100 percent. Most policies reimburse providers at 80 percent of the "usual, customary and reasonable" charge (meaning the going rate in your neck of the woods, which we'll discuss in greater detail a bit later).

The other 20 percent of your medical expenses (or whatever percent it is the policy won't cover if yours is not 80/20 coverage) is called your *coinsurance*. That's the money you have to pay out of your own pocket.

Speaking of that money coming out of your own pants, most policies (fortunately) have an *out-of-pocket* maximum. This means that once you've personally paid out this specified amount in coinsurance in a given year, the insurance company will cover the coinsurance for you for the rest of that year (for the "usual, customary and reasonable" expenses, that is).

Of course from the time you purchase your policy, you pay (or perhaps your employer pays for you) a monthly *premium* to continue its coverage. And you must also pay an annual *deductible*, another bit of money you have to pay out of your own pocket toward your medical expenses before your insurance will even begin to kick in on your behalf.

(One quick note: An *indemnity* policy is similar to a fee-for-service plan in that it pays per each service rendered, but it's different in that it pays the money to you and not to your provider. You then have the freedom to pay your doctor or hospital however you see fit.)

The upside to a fee-for-service plan is that you can pretty much choose whatever doctor or hospital you want. The downside is unfortunately a bit steeper. Fee-for-service plans:

- are **expensive**, when you consider the cost of the deductibles and coinsurance;
- can be terribly **hard to understand**, which can hurt especially when you're the one who has the responsibility to fill out the forms and keep track of the claims and make the payments; and they
- rarely cover **commonsense preventive measures** such as baby wellness visits and annual checkups.

MANAGED CARE COVERAGE

A managed care plan is an entirely different animal from a fee-for-service plan. Instead of paying fees to providers per each service rendered, managed care plans generally provide comprehensive health services to members in exchange for their choosing doctors and hospitals belonging to the plan. In other words, rather than waiting for a company to pay for each medical service as it comes along, you *prepay* a company to cover the costs of all the medical services you may ever need.

(And you thought that's what traditional insurance premiums were all about. It only seemed that way, you neophyte!)

Managed care comes in one of three forms: *health maintenance organizations* (HMOs), *preferred provider organizations* (PPOs), and *point-of-service* (POS) plans.

1) Health maintenance organizations (HMOs). With a health maintenance organization, you don't have to worry about paying deductibles and coinsurance. Generally, you pay only a *co-payment* for certain services, maybe $300 for a hospital stay or $10 for an office visit or $5 for every prescription. Everything else is covered fully—as long as you follow the proper procedures.

With most HMOs, you select a *primary care physician*—usually a family practitioner, a pediatrician, or an internist—who coordinates your entire medical care. Your primary care physician must refer you to any specialists you may need, and when he does, he will almost always refer you to a specialist who's also a participating provider within the HMO.

Some HMOs will deliver the care directly through a particular medical facility, while others will coordinate your care through a broader network of participating providers.

2) Preferred provider organizations (PPOs). A preferred provider organization offers its members managed care with a little bit more flexibility. A PPO is comprised of a network of doctors and hospitals who charge patients on a fee-for-service basis. Members usually pay deductibles and coinsurance. So a PPO is kind of like a hybrid between a standard HMO plan and a traditional fee-for-service plan.

The difference between a PPO and a standard HMO is this: You have the freedom to go outside the managed care network if you want and still receive some coverage. Also, you generally don't have to have a primary care physician coordinate your care. Unfortunately, you pay more for this freedom.

On the other hand, the difference between a PPO and a traditional fee-for-service plan is this: It's cheaper. When you go to a doctor or hospital within the network, you pay less in coinsurance for their services than you do when you go to a doctor or hospital outside the network.

3) Point-of-service (POS) plans. A point-of-service plan combines the cost-effectiveness of an HMO with the flexibility of a PPO. When you stay within the managed care network of participating providers, as with an HMO, you pay no deductibles or coinsurance for services rendered, and only a small co-pay for each hospital stay, doctor visit, or prescription. But when you choose to go outside the network of participating providers, as with a PPO, then you pay deductibles and coinsurance as part of your coverage.

The upside to a managed care plan is primarily twofold. Managed care coverage is cheaper than fee-for-service coverage. And it's also a lot easier to understand and manage. In its purer forms, there are no annual deductibles to calculate and pay, no claims to file, and no coinsurance to pay. Prescriptions are generally paid for. And, as alluded to earlier, managed care typically covers preventive care.

The downside is that managed care plans:

- may **limit your choice of doctors** to those within the network, whether you have to work through a primary care physician or not; and they
- may **limit your choice of medical services** to those deemed medically necessary by the HMO, PPO, or POS.

Both fee-for-service and managed care plans have negatives in addition to the ones we've mentioned here. We'll explore more of the underside of insurance coverage in the chapters that follow.

OTHER FORMS OF INSURANCE

In addition to these primary fee-for-service and managed care plans, health insurance is also available in other forms:

1) Medicare. Perhaps the best-known federal health insurance program, Medicare offers coverage to those citizens sixty-five years old and older and to the disabled who aren't covered by an employer. Medicare coverage comes in two forms: Medicare Part A covers hospitalization costs, while Medicare Part B covers physicians' services.

While we all contribute to the costs of Part A coverage through our Social Security taxes, Part B is a voluntary program supplemented through the monthly premiums of those who choose to participate.

Because Medicare can't cover all the charges a patient might incur, private companies offer what are known as *Medicare supplement policies* (sometimes called Medigap or MedSupp policies) to fill in the gaps. These policies are required to cover certain charges, such as the total deductible for a hospital stay and the remaining percentage of all Medicare-covered charges left unpaid after Medicare coverage has been exhausted.

Depending on geographic location, Medicare recipients may have a choice between fee-for-service and managed care plans.

2) Medicaid. Title XIX of the Social Security Act provides medical assistance for low-income individuals and families—Medicaid. The program was created in 1965, a year before Medicare first appeared. Medicaid is a joint federal-state health insurance program run by each state for its impoverished citizens (children and pregnant women in particular) and for its disabled. Some states now require their Medicaid recipients to join managed care plans.

3) Other governmental plans. The United States government also offers insurance coverage for military personnel past and present, for federal civilian employees, and for certain special-interest groups like the American Indians and Alaskan natives.

4) Long-term care insurance. Long-term care policies cover the high costs of long-term care—nursing home care, home health care, and long-term therapy—which typically are not covered by other insurance, save for Medicare (which will cover services rendered only at a certain level) and Medicaid.

Though few of us want to consider the possibility of a chronic illness or disability, financially speaking, more of us should. Basic nursing home care can run as much as $150 a day. That translates to over $50,000 per year! Skilled nursing care runs much higher. And pharmacy bills alone can run an additional $500–$600 per month. Just to have a home health aide come into your home three times a week to assist with bathing and dressing and such can cost you over $12,000 a year!

Long-term care insurance coverage isn't cheap. But it may be worth the cost.

5) Medical savings accounts. In 1996 Congress passed the Health Insurance Portability and Accountability Act (HIPAA), which created what are called medical savings accounts (MSAS). To be eligible for this type of coverage, a person must either be self-employed or work for a small employer (fifty or fewer employees) who offers an MSA plan.

Basically, an MSA allows you to make tax-deductible contributions to an account out of which you pay your health expenses. First you choose a fee-for-service plan from an insurance company, then you convert it into an MSA by paying a higher deductible in exchange for a (much) lower premium.

You deposit tax-free the difference between the normal fee-for-service premium and the substantially lowered MSA premium. Anytime you incur a medical expense, you just pay for it out of this account up to the amount at which your deductible is met (at which time, of course, your insurance kicks in). The healthier you stay, the more money you keep in your account.

(For further information about medical savings accounts or the Health Insurance Portability and Accountability Act, you can contact the Council for Affordable Health Insurance, 112 S. West St., Suite 400, Alexandria, VA 22314, [703] 836-6200.)

10

An Ounce of Prevention

HOW TO FIX SOME PROBLEMS BEFORE THEY ARISE

"Let's talk about the Black file," I say. "It was assigned to you."

"That's correct. The initial claim form from Mrs. Black was assigned to me. Pursuant to company policy at that time, I sent her a letter of denial."

"Why?"

"Why? Because all claims were initially denied, at least in 1991."

"All claims?"

"Yes. It was our policy to deny every claim initially, then review the smaller ones that appeared to be legitimate. We eventually paid some of those, but the big claims were never paid unless a lawyer got involved."

"But you knew the claim should be paid?"

"Everybody knew it, but the company was playing the odds."

"Could you explain this?"

"The odds that the insured wouldn't consult a lawyer."

"Did you know what the odds were at the time?"

"It was commonly believed that no more than one out of twenty-five would talk to a lawyer. That's the only reason they started this experiment. They knew they could get by with it. They sell these policies to people who are not that educated, and they count on their ignorance to accept the denials."

—*from* The Rainmaker, *by John Grisham*

The above courtroom dialogue is fiction. The company John Grisham described, Great Benefit Life Insurance Company, never existed. But similar to Great Benefit Life, real insurance companies and HMOs count on *your* ignorance to accept *their* denials.

In the next chapter we'll begin educating you on some of the things you can do to make sure your insurer "does what it says and says what it does" in regard to your claims. But since an ounce of prevention is worth a pound of cure, we'll look first at what you can do to fix the problems before they even begin. Let's consider what you should look for when *choosing* a health insurance plan.

After all, if you choose to buy a health insurance policy from a company like Great Benefit Life, how much good is it going to do you to haggle with them over a single claim?

HAVE IT YOUR WAY

Perhaps you've begun a new job and your employer offers you a choice of health insurance plans, or perhaps you have no opportunity for group coverage at all and you need to find an individual insurance plan to cover you and your family. How do you go about finding the right plan for you?

Fortunately, you can get a lot of the information you need without ever leaving the house. Using this book as a starting point, you can then use your computer and your telephone to learn just about everything you'll need.

1) Decide which type of coverage fits you best. Review the types of plans we laid out in chapter 9. Would your prefer a fee-for-service plan or a managed care plan? Do you want an HMO, a PPO, or a POS?

First, find out which plans are available to you in your area. Then determine which plan best fits your budget, your mental comfort level, and your health care needs.

Do you want to keep the doctor you have now? Call him and find out which plans he participates in. Do you want to go to the hospital down the street whenever you need care? Find out which plans they accept. You probably don't want to choose an insurance plan that excludes your doctor or hospital of choice, no matter how great it looks on paper.

2) Do the research. Detailed information about these different types of coverage—and, more important, about the specific companies that offer them—is easy to find.

The Internet is an invaluable tool in this regard. There are Web sites out there designed specifically to help consumers navigate the stormy waters of the insurance industry. Here are a few I highly recommend you check out:

- **www.insure.com** (Consumer Insurance Guide)
  This site combines "the reporting style of a daily newspaper with a wealth of up-to-date resource information." In addition to the latest insurance news, it offers insurance company guides, a complaint finder, a lawsuit library, a glossary, a link directory, and answers to frequently asked insurance questions.
- **www.hiaa.org** (Health Insurance Association of America)
  This site offers a host of good information, including detailed consumers' guides that explain in easy-to-understand terms various health insurance issues. At least one of the guides was developed in conjunction with the U.S. Department of Health and Human Services.
- **www.naic.org** (National Association of Insurance Commissioners)
  This site is geared more toward the insurance industry than toward consumers, but it does offer a variety of consumer booklets on specific health insurance topics as well as contact information for each state insurance commissioner.
- **www.hcfa.org** (Health Care Financing Administration)
  HCFA is the federal agency that administers the Medicare, Medicaid, and Child Health programs. For official information about any of these government plans, this is a good place to look.

Every state has an insurance commissioner whose office oversees the industry within his or her state. Call your state insurance commissioner's office and ask what resources they provide consumers.

And this is critical: Before you sign on with a particular company or plan, be sure to check its track record with your state insurance commissioner, who can tell you the number and the types of complaints that policyholders and plan members have leveled against that company.

3) Read your policy. I know it probably sounds about as appealing as a root canal, but you need to do it. Think of it this way: An hour or so of unpleasantness up front can save months of anguish down the road.

Don't get fooled into reading just the promotional literature an insurance company offers you. And don't just read the plan's summary of benefits. Read the *entire* policy, front to back. That's the only place the rubber actually hits the road, legally speaking.

YOU BETTER SHOP AROUND

According to insure.com, the National Association of Insurance Commissioners offers the following "Health Insurance Shopping Checklist," which I think offers advice worth considering when choosing a plan or reviewing a policy:

Coverage

- What does the plan pay for?
- What does the plan not pay for/exclude?
- What are the limits on preexisting medical conditions?
- Will the plan pay for preventive care, immunizations, well-baby care, substance abuse, organ transplants,

vision care, dental care, infertility treatment, durable medical equipment, or chiropractic care?

- Will the plan pay for prescriptions?
- Does the plan have mental health benefits?
- Will the plan pay for long-term physical therapy?

Premiums

- Do rates increase as you age?
- How often can rates be changed?
- How much do you have to pay when you receive health care services (co-payments and deductibles)?
- Are there any limits on how much you must pay for health care services you receive (out-of-pocket maximums)?
- Are there any limits on the number of times you may receive a service (lifetime maximums or annual benefit caps)?

Customer Service

- Has the company had an unusually high number of consumer complaints?
- What happens when you call the company's consumer complaint number?
- How long does it take to reach a real person?

"Think about your personal situation," counsels the Health Insurance Association of America. "After all, you may not mind that pregnancy is not covered; but you may want coverage for psychological counseling. Do you want coverage for your whole family or just yourself? Are you concerned with preventive care and checkups? Or would you be comfortable in a managed care setting that might restrict your choice somewhat but give you broad coverage and convenience? These are questions that only you can answer."

ACTION POINTS

❑ **Determine the type of insurance that's best for you.** First decide whether you want a fee-for-service plan or a managed care plan. If managed care is what you want, would you rather be a member of an HMO, a PPO, or a POS?

❑ **Determine the plan that's best for you.** Get on the Internet and do your homework. Make sure you understand the jargon insurance companies use and the issues that lie behind the jargon. Search out information on any specific companies you're considering buying from.

❑ **Contact your state insurance commissioner.** Call the insurance commissioner's office and request any help they can give you, whether it be literature on a certain topic or a history of consumer complaints against a company under your consideration.

❑ **Read through your entire insurance policy.** Get beyond the marketing materials and the summaries. Read the policy itself. It can be done. And you can do it. Remember, an hour or two of unpleasantness up front can save months of anguish down the road.

11

Heart Failure

How to Recognize and Reverse Insurance Denials, Part I

March 4, 1998

Dear Pat and Martha,

Here's the final payment (I think) on my bill.

Again, thank you both so much! You are a Godsend to someone wrapped up in fighting for their life and having to worry about finances as well.

I've given your names to lots of people.

Regards, your Big Fan,

Kim

This was one of the last notes I ever received from Kimberly Neumann.

I was as much a fan of her as she was of me. Kim was a businesswoman in my hometown who had enjoyed an award-winning career in newspaper journalism before she ran an award-winning public relations and advertising firm.

The forty-six-year-old mother of three was by nature a winner, and that was a good thing.

Because while Kim was already fighting the biggest fight of her life against cancer, she found herself forced into a fight against her insurance company as well. Ultimately, after a long, hard-fought battle, the cancer finally overcame her.

But at least the insurance company didn't.

This is her story.

Kim was a member of a PPO plan offered by one of the nation's best-known insurers. Over the two-and-a-half-year course of her medical treatment, she saw more than thirty-nine different providers.

One provider was a highly esteemed university hospital in a neighboring state. Their finance department harassed her unmercifully whenever she came in for treatments. They wanted $4,000 from her.

"Talk to my insurance company!" she kept telling them.

Under the terms of her managed care agreement, she had a $2,000 annual out-of-pocket limit. So how on earth could she possibly owe them $4,000?

The hospital didn't offer any firm answers. The only thing they seemed to know was that Kim's PPO had denied $4,000 worth of treatments and services. And they wanted their money.

And so the battle raged on, and not just with that provider, but with others as well. Even with her $2,000 out-of-pocket limit, Kim was somehow left holding a bag full of bills worth over $20,000!

Twenty thousand dollars! More than *ten times* her out-of-pocket limit!

What had gone wrong?

As we investigated, it became obvious that many things had. Some services that clearly were supposed to have been covered had been denied coverage. Sometimes a provider had attached an incorrect code to a particular service. Other times the date of service had simply been mistyped.

The primary problem with her bill turned out to be the rate at which certain providers had been reimbursed. Again and again and again, the services of *participating* providers had been reimbursed as if they had been *nonparticipating* providers. Among other reasons, Kim's PPO claimed her records didn't indicate she had gotten the proper referrals her plan required. So rather than receiving 80 percent coverage for many services, Kim received only 60 percent coverage—and an alarming amount of outright denials to boot.

The scariest part of this story is that Kim actually did do all the right things. She worked diligently with her primary care physician. She went through the proper channels and got the proper referrals she needed to see all the specialists her care required.

But still things went terribly awry.

Little things. Dumb things. But enough to make Kim's "out-of-pocket" obligation skyrocket to over $20,000.

Together, we were able to overcome her "managed care" mess. After doing the necessary research, and then pointing out to Kim's PPO the errors of their ways, they agreed to cover almost the entire $20,000.

As they should have from the beginning.

What was Kim Neumann's final, accurate "out-of-pocket" payment? Eighteen hundred dollars—two hundred dollars *less* than her out-of-pocket maximum as stated in her policy.

Kim Neumann spent the last years of her life worrying about having to pay medical bills her managed care plan should have paid from day one, at a time when she needed every bit of strength and every bit of willpower she could muster to focus on the cancer eating away at her body.

She had played by the rules. She had done all the right things. And still her bills haunted her to the end.

DOOMSDAY SCENARIOS

What if Kim Neumann hadn't been able to resolve her insurance company's foibles? Or what if she had been able to, but not within a time frame acceptable to the providers who were after her to pay the money?

By the time we were finally able to resolve Kim's insurance coverage, her bills were almost ten months past due. One of the providers was only days away from sending her bills to a collection agency.

What would have happened then?

Her credit report, of course, would have reflected her delinquency. She probably would have been harassed with phone calls and letters from the collection agency. If she had wanted to buy a home, she probably would have been denied a loan. And she probably would have had to pay thousands of dollars just to have her credit record "cleared" of debt she never even owed in the first place.

What else could have happened?

The providers could have just refused to treat her anymore, due to her inability to pay.

Anything else?

Well, consider the case of Martha Ellis's mother. Martha's mom, like mine, contracted cancer, but her mother's treatment required three shots a week at a cost of $795 per shot—for two years.

The clinic she went to actively pursues delinquent bills after sixty days, at which point they also begin tacking on interest charges. For one reason or another, Medicare kept denying Martha's mother's claims for two years, and her bills grew to $90,000—plus $3,000 more in interest.

If Martha hadn't been there to reassure her father along the way that in fact he didn't owe the clinic this money out of his own pocket, she and I both know exactly what he would have done.

He would have sold his house to make the payment. That's the kind of man he is.

We'd like to think that these scenarios never actually play out in real life. Unfortunately, they do. All the time. This sort of thing happens all across America every day of the week.

GOING FOR BROKE

Why is it that doctors and hospitals turn so quickly to their patients' pockets for payment when an insurance claim is denied?

Frankly, because the payoff—if they can get it—is *bigger*.

Insurance companies (both fee-for-service and managed care companies) always negotiate lower rates with doctors and hospitals. They pay less for services, goods, and procedures than what the general public has to pay. For example, an X ray that costs you $80 might in fact cost your insurer only $60! A chemotherapy treatment that costs you $500 might cost your insurer only $250.

That means that if you have a fee-for-service insurer who agrees to cover that X ray under a standard 80/20 policy, they will pay $48 of their negotiated $60 fee and you will pay the remaining 20 percent coinsurance of $12.

Easy enough?

But hold on. If they choose to *deny* the claim, then you'll have to pay $80 out-of-pocket, not the $60 your insurer would have paid. It only gets worse. Since your insurer won't cover the charge, it doesn't fall under the jurisdiction the out-of-pocket limit stated on your policy.

Or let's imagine you're a member of an HMO, and they agree to cover that chemotherapy treatment. In that case, they might pay the entire negotiated fee of $250, and you'd pay nothing. But should they happen to *reject* the claim—perhaps by challenging its "medical necessity"—don't expect the hospital to accept $250 from *you* as payment in full. At that point they're going to ask for the full retail price of $500.

Sound fair?

Hardly, when you consider how stingy the insurers (HMOs in particular) have become about paying for services and treatments that were once considered routine.

LEGAL RECOURSE

In fact, class-action lawsuits against HMOs have made big headlines in recent months, as people are now turning to the courts to seek remedy from companies who have provided what they consider to be shabby managed care treatment.

Five of the industry's biggest companies—CIGNA Corporation, Foundation Health Systems Inc., Humana Inc., PacifiCare, and The Prudential Insurance Company of America—were recently sued for violating the Civil Racketeer Influenced and Corrupt Organizations Act (RICO) and the Employee Retirement Security Income Act (ERISA).

They were sued by the same group of lawyers who went after the tobacco companies (using the same legal strategy). Richard Scruggs, the group's lead attorney, said at the time the actions were filed, "We're acting today to fix the broken promises the HMO industry has made to the people who entrust their very lives to these companies. We will ensure that MDs—not MBAs or CPAs—will determine patient treatment.

"The plague of HMOs telling enrollees their physical health matters most while putting corporate financial health first has infected all these companies," he went on to say. "Our lawsuits will heal this industry through a simple prescription: Do what you say and say what you do."

This group had already made headlines by similarly suing the largest HMO in the nation, Aetna U.S. Healthcare.

There's a reason such lawsuits are suddenly popping up across the nation: In October 1999, the U.S. House of Representatives passed a bipartisan Patients' Bill of Rights, which for the first time gave HMO members the right to sue their HMO. (At the time of this writing, the bill has not passed in the Senate.)

I believe that this legislation is a much-needed step in the right direction.

Not surprisingly, HMOs (and other health insurers) say

it's not. They argue that the lawyers doing the suing are only interested in lining their own pockets, which may be partially true.

But patients still need a way to make their voices heard.

The HMOs claim they already offer an effective way for patients to make themselves heard: a formal appeals process that allows dissatisfied members to challenge company decisions, either to the HMO directly or (in some states) to an external review board. HMOs say that the cost of defending themselves against these newly approved lawsuits will only result in higher premiums for patients.

I don't doubt that for a minute, given that insurers raise premium rates at the drop of a hat. But just ask someone like Cynthia Herdich of Illinois if patients deserve the right to sue.

While a member of an HMO called Alliance Health Medical Plans in the early 1990s, Ms. Herdich was forced to wait eight days for approval of a sonogram to verify whether or not she was suffering from appendicitis.

While she was waiting for that approval to come, her appendix burst.

Ms. Herdrich sued her doctor, clinic, and HMO for damages, saying that the physician-owned company had a conflicting financial incentive to deny claims over patients' needs. The trial court initially dismissed the case against the HMO, but following an appeal by Ms. Herdich, the case is being reconsidered.

In another case, somewhat similar to that of my late friend Kim Neumann, a woman appealed to Anthem Blue Cross and Blue Shield to pay for cancer treatments they spuriously denied as "experimental."

Did she get justice from her HMO's appeals process? Hardly. By the time the process was over, she was dead.

Her widowed husband sued—and was awarded $51.5 million.

The bottom line for patients is this: We're getting squeezed on both ends. On one end we get squeezed by our providers, and on the other end we get squeezed by our insurers! Insurance companies routinely deny patient claims they ought to cover, and doctors and hospitals prematurely bill their patients for that money, hoping for bigger, quicker payouts.

This is the world we've created.

ACTION POINTS

☐ **Expect to pay more than your out-of-pocket limit.** Your out-of-pocket maximum only applies to those charges your insurance company agrees to cover. Any claim they deny—or, as we'll see later, any *portion* of a claim they deny—is money that comes out of your pocket, no matter what the limit is on your policy.

☐ **Expect to pay retail prices for non-covered expenses.** If a claim is denied, you'll probably have to pay more for that service or item than your insurance company would have—sometimes a lot more. Be prepared for that $250 chemotherapy treatment to jump to $500 once it becomes your responsibility.

☐ **Don't pay any "bills" from your doctors or hospital until your insurance situation is resolved.** These are just blatant attempts to get you to pay money you don't owe. Don't sell the house. Wait for resolution from your insurance company, no matter how long it takes.

☐ **Make sure your insurer pays all claims at the right rate.** Double-check your claim statements to make sure your managed care network is reimbursing as they should—and not claiming that you went out of network or failed to get a referral when in fact you "did all the right things."

☐ **Argue your case.** Take advantage of your insurer's appeals process. If that doesn't work to your satisfaction, the courts are now available.

12

Compound Fractures

HOW TO RECOGNIZE AND REVERSE INSURANCE DENIALS, PART II

"What caused the death of Donny Ray Black?"

He shrugs. "Leukemia."

"And what medical condition prompted the filing of his claim?"

"Leukemia."

"In your letter there, what preexisting condition do you mention?"

"The flu."

"And when did he have the flu?"

"I think he was fifteen or sixteen," he says.

"So he had the flu when he was fifteen or sixteen, before the policy was issued, and this was not mentioned on the application."

"That's correct."

"Now, Mr. Pellrod, in your vast experience in claims, have you ever seen a case in which a bout with the flu was somehow related to the onset of acute leukemia five years later?"

There's only one answer, but he just can't give it. "I don't think so."

"So you lied in your letter, didn't you?"

"The letter was a mistake," Pellrod says.

"A mistake that helped kill Donny Ray Black?"

I turn and point to Dot Black, then look at the witness. "Mr. Pellrod, as the senior claims examiner, can you look Mrs. Black squarely in the eyes and tell her that her son's claim was handled fairly by your office? Can you do this?"

He squints and twitches and frowns, and glances at [his lawyer] for instructions. He clears his throat, tries to act offended, says, "I don't believe I can be forced to do that."

"Thank you. No further questions."

—abridged excerpt from The Rainmaker,
by John Grisham

I just couldn't resist adding one more piece of courtroom drama from John Grisham. It may sound ridiculous to some that an insurance claim for leukemia could be rejected due to a preexisting bout with the flu, but the fact of the matter is, life really does imitate Grisham's art.

Real-life insurance companies sometimes pull the same kind of stunt that the fictitious Great Benefit Life Insurance company pulled.

Sometimes they succeed. And sometimes they don't.

PREEXISTING NONSENSE

Consider this stranger-than-fiction case.

In September of 1996 Lillian Craft was diagnosed with

a toxic thyroid condition. She received treatments for the problem over the course of several months that followed. All the while, she was insured through an HMO plan her husband's company provided.

In March of the following year, Lillian received the following disturbing notice from a financial counselor at her hospital: "We regret to inform you that your insurance company has denied benefits for this claim for the reason stated above."

The reason stated above? "CLAIM DENIED AS PREEXISTING."

The hospital asked that Lillian remit payment to them for the balance of all the treatments within thirty days.

She turned to us for help.

Unlike Great Benefit, Lillian's HMO had found a legitimate thyroid treatment in her medical history. It was a thyroid lobectomy, performed for less than $500 as an outpatient operation.

It would have been just cause for "preexisting condition" denial in anybody's book—except that it happened in 1981. The operation had been absolutely successful. It had been followed by no special therapy and no type of drug maintenance. For over fifteen years, Lillian had not experienced even *one* thyroid problem.

We asked the HMO to justify their classifying this as a preexisting condition after fifteen trouble-free years. In a letter to Lillian, they responded:

"Based on the questions you completed when your husband requested that you be added to his coverage, it stated you already had problems with a thyroid condition. Our plan has a pre-existing clause that states if a condition, illness, or injury has its origin to any degree, whether diagnosed or not, prior to their effective date of coverage, no claims will be paid for a period of five years.

"By your own admission this condition fit the preexisting clause. This is the reason for the claims being denied."

They deemed it a preexisting condition because *Lillian* had said it was. Forget that she just filled out a question on their application form in the only way it could be answered; you'd think she had reluctantly admitted to committing a grave criminal offense.

Actually, their primary defense was the language of their less-than-generous preexisting clause: So long as Lillian's condition had its origin prior to her date of coverage *to any degree*, it was "preexisting."

So, according to their policy, she could have had thyroid surgery in an eighteenth-century past life. If she'd had it ever—*to any degree*—it wouldn't be covered until five years after the date her coverage began.

I thought this was highly suspicious, and so did the investigator with the Labor Department's Pension and Welfare Benefits Administration office, to whom I had gone for help after the company turned downright belligerent.

Lo and behold, soon after being contacted by the investigator, the HMO reconsidered its decision. It decided to pay Lillian's claims after all.

Heck, come to find out, they had actually changed that preexisting clause—limiting its duration to just eighteen months—way back in September of 1996, at about the same time Lillian's claims had first begun!

The HMO's explanation? "The claims processor who handled the claims was under the impression that only new employees hired after September 1996 would fall under the new guidelines," they told Lillian in a letter, which also happened to contain their sincerest apologies.

Golly. So it had all been just one big misunderstanding? It was just . . . a *mistake?*

Thank you, no further questions.

(Fortunately, the government has since tightened preexisting condition clauses considerably. According to current law, insurance companies can only impose a *twelve-month* waiting period for any preexisting condition treated or diagnosed within *six months* prior to the start of coverage.)

QUESTION EVERYTHING

If the above stories teach you anything, the lesson should be to *question everything*.

Don't ever accept an insurance company's denial of coverage at face value. Not every company is out to defraud you. Many denials are legitimate. But claims are handled by people, and people will always make mistakes—especially when they're poorly trained and have no formal medical knowledge on which to base their decisions.

Understand this lesson and learn it well: Erroneous hospital overcharges are no worse than erroneous insurance company denials. That's a scary thought, I know, it's true.

Hospitals and insurance companies get you coming and going . . . so question everything.

RETAIL VS. WHOLESALE

Not long ago, someone sent me some excerpts from a hospital administration textbook called *The Financial Man-*

agement of Hospitals that offer an insider's glance into how hospital pricing is decided. Here are a couple excerpts:

"Hospital managers have traditionally had to view pricing as an issue solely for their relationships with self-insured patients or commercial insurance payers who could not strike a special pricing arrangement with the hospital."

So too bad for you if you're uninsured or insured by an insurance company with no clout. Why?

"These patients [the properly insured], in effect, pay for care at cost or slightly above cost, while self-insured patients pay for care on the basis of charges that are dictated by financial expediency, that is, charges established at levels designed to generate revenues equal to cost plus whatever additional funds are needed to meet the hospital's financial requirements."

In other words, while they're being negotiated down by insurance companies, hospitals are forced to make up the difference on the backs of the self-insured and poorly insured.

While the insurance companies pay wholesale, Joe Q. Public pays retail. Pity the poor people—about seventy million of them in all, recent reports indicate—who don't have adequate insurance and have to pay full retail prices.

CRUEL AND UNUSUAL

Even when you have insurance coverage and your insurance company agrees to cover your claims, you still may not be out of the woods. Remember, what the insurance company offers to pay may not match up with what the doctor or hospital wants to charge.

When that happens, as it often does, guess who pays the difference?

You do, of course . . . and me.

How does that work?

Earlier we saw that fee-for-service insurance companies typically cover 80 percent of accepted medical charges. But that doesn't guarantee they'll cover 80 percent of the total price you've been charged for a service. It only guarantees they'll cover 80 percent of what *they* consider a "usual, customary and reasonable" charge.

What does *that* mean?

Insurance companies determine the price they'll pay for a given service based on the going rate, on what other doctors (or therapists or equipment wholesalers or whoever) are charging for that service in your area. If your doctor's charge falls below that "usual, customary and reasonable" rate, you're in the clear.

But if he charges *more* than what they think he should— unless your doctor has agreement with your insurer to write off such costs—*you* have to pay the difference. Unfortunately, it happens all the time: Patients are forced to pay money out of their own pockets for claims their insurance companies approve, but won't pay fully.

Again, this is money not included in your out-of-pocket limit. This is money the hospital expects you to pay, no matter how high it piles up.

Finding out what an insurance company considers to be "usual, customary and reasonable" isn't always easy. The information can be had, but most of us probably aren't going to take the time and effort necessary to figure out how much our insurer will reimburse for a given service *before* that service is rendered.

However, in the case of a major surgery or an expensive piece of durable medical equipment, *ask* your insurer what they consider "usual, customary and reasonable."

EXCEPTIONAL SERVICE

One thing I do recommend is to check out the exceptions to each item that's listed in your policy's benefits summary. This simple step can help keep you from paying money you don't owe.

For example, let's say your policy calls for a $100 annual deductible. Before you pay, read the details about your deductible listed under the exceptions.

You may find you don't have to pay the deductible in the case of an accident. Or maybe you don't have to pay another $100 at the beginning of the calendar year if you just paid it during the last three months of the year before. Or maybe only three out of the five members of your family are required to pay the deductible.

This is just one example.

But keep an eye out for the exceptions for all your benefits, because if you don't, I guarantee, no one else will.

FINDERS KEEPERS

Not all the news is bad news. Believe it or not, you can make money off of bad medical bills even if your insurance company covers every last dime of your medical expenses!

How? In at least one of two ways.

First, medical billing has become such a mess that insurance companies are now paying rewards to policyholders and plan members to help them stop the nonsense.

If you find errors in your hospital bill, some insurance companies will pay you one-half of the money you save them. Check your insurance booklet to see if your insurance company has such a policy. If their policy is not stated, call them and ask.

And secondly, federal whistle-blower laws, which allow individual employees to sue companies on behalf of the government, can be quite lucrative. Medical and insurance workers who bring such suits can reap rewards as high as 15 to 30 percent of the amount the government recovers.

Several people associated with Columbia/HCA Health care Corp. secretly filed these types of lawsuits against the company back in 1997, allowing the government to build its case against Columbia/HCA for Medicare fraud.

Somehow I'm not surprised that the fastest growing industry for such suits is reported to be the health care industry.

ACTION POINTS

❏ **Question everything.** Never let a denied claim pass by uncontested. Claims are handled by people, and people make mistakes. And, sometimes, believe it or not, people can be devious.

❏ **Find out what's "usual, customary and reasonable."** In the case of a major surgery, treatment, or an expensive piece of durable medical equipment, make sure you know how much your insurance company will pay—ahead of time.

❏ **Check the exceptions.** To keep from paying money you don't owe, read the details behind every item listed on your insurance policy's summary of benefits. If you don't spot the exceptions, no one else will.

❏ **Blow the whistle.** If you spot errors in your medical bill, check to see if your insurance company will reward you for the effort. Many do, sometimes paying half of what they recover. Check your insurance booklet for your insurer's policy. If you can't find one, call the company and ask.

13

The Road to Recovery

A STEP-BY-STEP PRESCRIPTION

REGARDING YOUR DOCTOR AND
HOSPITAL BILLS . . .

Step One

- **Wake up!** Times have changed. Hospitals aren't billing straight, and insurers aren't reimbursing straight. You shouldn't allow yourself to get squeezed between a health care system that *was* and a health care system that *is*.

- **Refuse to be bullied.** Resolve not to allow yourself to be pressured by any health care provider into paying money you don't owe.

- **Refuse to pay as you go.** Don't be duped into believing you have to pay off your bill before you leave the hospital or clinic following a major procedure. Remember, it's much too early for anyone to tell you how much is really owed at this point, much less who's responsible for payment.

Step Two

- **Get a real bill.** Recognize the difference between a summary bill and an itemized bill. Should your hospital or doctor send you a summary bill with only categories of charges listed (which they probably will), ask them to give you an itemized bill that details every specific expense you have incurred.

- **Refuse to take no for an answer.** Should a hospital or doctor in any way try to avoid giving you an itemized bill, remind them politely yet firmly that they must do so under penalty of state law. Tell them that no matter how strange a request they think it is, no matter how much insurance you have, no matter where the bill has been "sent," no matter how little or how much you've already paid, they are required to give you an itemized bill. Ask to talk to a manager when necessary.

- **Keep itemizing.** Get itemized bills too from any health care professionals who happen to bill you separately following a major medical procedure.

- **Take control.** Remember that the only person watching out for your interests is *you*—not your hospital, not your doctor, and not your insurance carrier or health maintenance organization.

- **If necessary, get help.** Find someone to review your bills for you if you cannot or do not want to do it yourself.

Step Three

- **If you don't know what something means, ask!**
  Don't let the foreign-sounding language of "medicalspeak" deter you. Be curious—it's your right and
  your responsibility.
- **Don't lose heart.** While the sight of your itemized
  medical bill may make you want to run for cover,
  don't. It's not as bad as it looks.
- **Order your medical records.** Send a brief written
  request to the medical records department of your
  hospital. Check with them first to find out what fees
  (retrieval and copying) they will charge. Make sure
  their charges are within the legal limits of the state.
- **Get help.** Call. Read. Ask. Be polite, yet firm.

Step Four

- **Take the lead.** Don't expect the government or your
  insurance company or your HMO to deflate the inflated prices on your medical bill. There's no law preventing the exaggerated prices. The responsibility is
  yours alone.
- **Compare prices.** You do it when you're buying a
  car. You do it when you're buying groceries. You
  should do it when you're buying medical care. Even
  if you failed to shop around before buying, comparing prices after the fact can still reap rewards. Knowledge is power.
- **Especially for big-ticket items, call your hospital's
  purchasing department to find out from whom
  they're buying.** That way you can find out exactly
  what they're paying. You don't need to tell the pur-

chasing agent that you're investigating the charges on your hospital bill. Let them know it's vital you get the information, but let them guess as to the reason why. (Maybe you need to purchase another one just like the one you've already bought?)

- **Call suppliers directly.** Ask them how much they charge. Do they offer discounts to hospitals? Bulk rates? What's their lowest price?
- **Leverage what you know.** Sit down with the financial director of your hospital and kindly yet firmly share the difference between their asking prices and the costs they actually paid. Remember, they'd rather negotiate and have you keep your information to yourself than risk others finding out. Even if they won't budge on some items, you'll still have added leverage in your favor when you discuss other problem areas with them, such as duplicate and hidden charges.
- **Be polite.** Remember, if you want honey, it does you no good at all to kick over the beehive.

Step Five

- **Unwrap the bundles.** If you find that a particular term on your bill refers to a bundled test or procedure, find out exactly what items are included in that bundle and check to make sure none of those items reappear elsewhere on your bill as a separate charge.
- **Disassemble the packages.** When you come across a "tray," a "package," or a "pack," you need to ensure that none of the items included in that package are also being charged separately.

- **Decline all extraneous photos.** When you come upon radiology charges, make sure the radiology department isn't charging you for some of their mistakes.
- **Unveil the mystery doctors.** When you get a bill from a "doctor you've never heard of," you need to find out who he was and what specific services he actually provided. How? Call him. Ask him. Make him show you some documentation. (Remember, if a service wasn't documented, it wasn't done.) Did the mystery doctor just pop his head in your room for a moment? Then challenge his charge. Did he serve as an assistant to your surgeon during surgery? Then make sure he isn't charging you any more than 20 percent of the fee you're paying your primary surgeon.

Step Six

- **Overturn all the scientific-sounding rocks.** Remember our commonsense rule from chapter 4: if you don't know what something means, ask. Some ridiculous charges can be hiding behind innocuous-sounding descriptions, and it's up to you to uncover the hidden meanings. Otherwise, items like "oral administration fees" and "cough support devices" could pile up on you.
- **Make sure you aren't paying a price for the constant use of an item that was only prescribed "as needed."** Remember, an oxygen "as needed" order can be detrimental to your financial health—even if you never actually used any oxygen. Check also for related charges incurred by any therapist or lab worker.

- **Don't get "stuck" paying for services that you've already paid for.** Venipuncture charges and "oral administration fees" are prime examples. You do not need to pay for nursing services that should be covered under the umbrella charge of your room rate.
- **Transport fees.** If you've paid $20 or $30 or more just for someone to carry your test tubes down the hall, then your bloodwork wasn't the only thing that got taken! Make sure your lab work was actually transported somewhere before you agree to pay any type of transport fee.

Step Seven

- **Don't get tagged with someone else's stickers.** While you're still in the hospital, if you can, have someone keep a watchful eye out for those little yellow stickers. Have them make sure your nurse doesn't mistakenly give you a little yellow sticker that happens to belong to another patient.
- **Create a Hospital Log.** Balance whatever has been ordered by your doctor against everything that actually was done.
- **If it wasn't documented, don't pay for it.** You don't have to pay for any item, service, or procedure that's not clearly documented as having been given or done in your medical records.
- **If it wasn't ordered, don't pay for it.** On the other hand, no matter what a nurse, therapist, technician, or anyone else has documented as having been done for you, if your doctor never ordered it, you are not responsible for paying for it. That goes for services, procedures, and supplies.

- **Balance your Hospital Log against your hospital bill.** Were you charged for services ordered but never performed? Were services performed that were never ordered? Check your hospital bill to see if you were charged for any of these possible errors.
- **Have your hospital billing department reconcile the differences.** Make them either provide the documentation you've found lacking or remove the charge. Remember, it's as simple as one, two, three. Don't expect them to put up much of a fight when you present them with cold hard facts!

REGARDING YOUR INSURANCE COVERAGE...

Step One

- **Determine the type of insurance that's best for you.** First decide whether you want a fee-for-service plan or a managed care plan. If managed care is what you want, would you rather be a member of an HMO, a PPO, or a POS?
- **Determine the plan that's best for you.** Get on the Internet and do your homework. Make sure you understand the jargon insurance companies use and the issues that lie behind the jargon. Search out information on any specific companies you're considering buying from.
- **Contact your state insurance commissioner.** Call the insurance commissioner's office and request any help they can give you, whether it be literature on a certain topic or a history of consumer complaints against a company under your consideration.

- **Read through your entire insurance policy.** Get beyond the marketing materials and the summaries. Read the policy itself. It can be done. And you can do it. Remember, an hour or two of unpleasantness up front can save months of anguish down the road.

Step Two

- **Expect to pay more than your out-of-pocket limit.** Your out-of-pocket maximum only applies to those charges your insurance company agrees to cover. Any claim they deny—or, as we have seen, any *portion* of a claim they deny—is money that comes out of your pocket, no matter what the limit is on your policy.

- **Expect to pay retail prices for noncovered expenses.** If a claim is denied, you'll probably have to pay more for that service or item than your insurance company would have—sometimes a lot more. Be prepared for that $250 chemotherapy treatment to jump to $500 once it becomes your responsibility.

- **Don't pay any "bills" from your doctors or hospital until your insurance situation is resolved.** These are just blatant attempts to get you to pay money you don't owe. Don't sell the house. Wait for resolution from your insurance company, no matter how long it takes.

- **Make sure your insurer pays all claims at the right rate.** Double-check your claim statements to make sure your managed care network is reimbursing as they should—and not claiming that you went out of network or failed to get a referral when in fact you "did all the right things."

- **Argue your case.** Take advantage of your insurer's appeals process. If that doesn't work to your satisfaction, the courts are now available.

Step Three

- **Question everything.** Never let a denied claim pass by uncontested. Claims are handled by people, and people make mistakes. And some people, believe it or not, can be devious.
- **Find out what's "usual, customary and reasonable."** In the case of a major surgery, treatment, or an expensive piece of durable medical equipment, make sure you know how much your insurance company will pay—ahead of time.
- **Check the exceptions.** To keep from paying money you don't owe, read the details behind every item listed on your insurance policy's summary of benefits. If you don't spot the exceptions, no one else will.
- **Blow the whistle.** If you spot errors in your medical bill, check to see if your insurance company will reward you for the effort. Many do, sometimes paying half of what they recover. Check your insurance booklet for your insurer's policy. If you can't find one, call the company and ask.

14

Preventive Medicine
TOWARD A PATIENT'S FINANCIAL BILL OF RIGHTS

"**C**onsumers and taxpayers are being nickeled and dimed out of, literally, billions of dollars each year—often with bilks so small that consumers think it is 'not worth the bother,'" charges consumer advocate Ralph Nader. "Also, many bills are either so vague or so inscrutably coded that it is impossible for the consumer to detect the overcharge."

Which industry does Ralph Nader consider to be the worst offender?

"Hospital billing errors are both the most common and the most grievous, in their size and their impact upon the elderly and poor," Nader says.

A simple glance at your own medical bills tells you that Nader is right. Medical billing, as it's currently practiced, is nothing short of criminal. Our bills *are* vague, inscrutably coded, and "grievous in their impact." Patients *are* being nickeled and dimed out of tons of money.

That being the case, every patient needs to know his or her rights. Yes, believe it or not, according to the American Hospital Association (AHA), we do have some rights. In 1973 they even adopted what they called "A Patient's Bill of Rights" (revised in 1992). A copy of the AHA's bill of rights follows.

However, there's a problem with this bill of rights: It doesn't go far enough. It only indirectly applies to medical billing. I strongly believe we deserve from our hospitals and insurance companies another bill of rights specific to the ethical treatment of patients as *consumers*.

I propose an additional bill of rights, one I call "A Patient's *Financial* Bill of Rights." I'd like to see the American Hospital Association—or better still, the Congress of the United States—adopt this simple bill for our protection.

My proposed bill of financial rights follows the patient's rights as currently spelled out by the American Hospital Association. As you read it alongside our currently promised rights, I hope you'll take careful note of the added protections it gives.

"We need 'truth in billing' legislation to provide consumers with the necessary tools for challenging erroneous bills," Ralph Nader said recently in defense of his legislative proposal for general billing reform. "Consumers need clear, itemized bills, and when they receive an erroneous bill, the burden should be on the company issuing the bill to justify the disputed charges."

"A Patient's Bill of Rights"

from the American Hospital Association
(www.aha.org/resource/pbillofrights.html)

INTRODUCTION

Effective health care requires collaboration between patients and physicians and other health care professionals. Open and honest communication, respect for personal and professional values, and sensitivity to differences are integral to optimal patient care. As the setting for the provision of health services, hospitals must provide a foundation for understanding and respecting the rights and responsibilities of patients, their families, physicians, and other caregivers. Hospitals must ensure a health care ethic that respects the role of patients in decision making about treatment choices and other aspects of their care. Hospitals must be sensitive to cultural, racial, linguistic, religious, age, gender, and other differences as well as the needs of persons with disabilities.

The American Hospital Association presents A Patient's Bill of Rights with the expectation that it will contribute to more effective patient care and be supported by the hospital on behalf of the institution, its medical staff, employees, and patients. The American Hospital Association encourages health care institutions to tailor this bill of rights to their patient community by translating and/or simplifying the language of this bill of rights as may be necessary to ensure that patients and their families understand their rights and responsibilities.

BILL OF RIGHTS

These rights can be exercised on the patient's behalf by a designated surrogate or proxy decision maker if the patient lacks decision-making capacity, is legally incompetent, or is a minor.

1. The patient has the right to considerate and respectful care.

2. The patient has the right to and is encouraged to obtain from physicians and other direct caregivers relevant, current, and understandable information concerning diagnosis, treatment, and prognosis.

    Except in emergencies when the patient lacks decision-making capacity and the need for treatment is urgent, the patient is entitled to the opportunity to discuss and request information related to the specific procedures and/or treatments, the risks involved, the possible length of recuperation, and the medically reasonable alternatives and their accompanying risks and benefits.

Patients have the right to know the identity of physicians, nurses, and others involved in their care, as well as when those involved are students, residents, or other trainees. The patient also has the right to know the immediate and long-term financial implications of treatment choices, insofar as they are known.

3. The patient has the right to make decisions about the plan of care prior to and during the course of treatment and to refuse a recommended treatment or plan of care to the extent permitted by law and hospital policy and to be informed of the medical consequences of this action. In case of such refusal, the patient is entitled to other appropriate care and services that the hospital provides or transfer to another hospital. The hospital should notify patients of any policy that might affect patient choice within the institution.

4. The patient has the right to have an advance directive (such as a living will, health care proxy, or durable power of attorney for health care) concerning treatment or designating a surrogate decision maker with the expectation that the hospital will honor the intent of that directive to the extent permitted by law and hospital policy.

Health care institutions must advise patients of their rights under state law and hospital policy to make informed medical choices, ask if the patient has an advance directive, and include that information in patient records. The patient has the right to timely information about hospital policy that may limit its ability to implement fully a legally valid advance directive.

5. The patient has the right to every consideration of privacy. Case discussion, consultation, examination, and treatment should be conducted so as to protect each patient's privacy.

6. The patient has the right to expect that all communications and records pertaining to his/her care will be treated as confidential by the hospital, except in cases such as suspected abuse and public health hazards when reporting is permitted or required by law. The patient has the right to expect that the hospital will emphasize the confidentiality of this information when it releases it to any other parties entitled to review information in these records.

7. The patient has the right to review the records pertaining to his/her medical care and to have the information explained or interpreted as necessary, except when restricted by law.

8. The patient has the right to expect that, within its capacity and policies, a hospital will make reasonable response to the request of a patient for appropriate and medically indicated care and services. The hospital must provide evaluation, service, and/or referral as indicated by the urgency of the case. When medically appropriate

and legally permissible, or when a patient has so requested, a patient may be transferred to another facility. The institution to which the patient is to be transferred must first have accepted the patient for transfer. The patient must also have the benefit of complete information and explanation concerning the need for, risks, benefits, and alternatives to such a transfer.

9. The patient has the right to ask and be informed of the existence of business relationships among the hospital, educational institutions, other health care providers, or payers that may influence the patient's treatment and care.

10. The patient has the right to consent to or decline to participate in proposed research studies or human experimentation affecting care and treatment or requiring direct patient involvement, and to have those studies fully explained prior to consent. A patient who declines to participate in research or experimentation is entitled to the most effective care that the hospital can otherwise provide.

11. The patient has the right to expect reasonable continuity of care when appropriate and to be informed by physicians and other caregivers of available and realistic patient care options when hospital care is no longer appropriate.

12. The patient has the right to be informed of hospital policies and practices that relate to patient

care, treatment, and responsibilities. The patient has the right to be informed of available resources for resolving disputes, grievances, and conflicts, such as ethics committees, patient representatives, or other mechanisms available in the institution. The patient has the right to be informed of the hospital's charges for services and available payment methods.

The collaborative nature of health care requires that patients, or their families/surrogates, participate in their care. The effectiveness of care and patient satisfaction with the course of treatment depend, in part, on the patient fulfilling certain responsibilities. Patients are responsible for providing information about past illnesses, hospitalizations, medications, and other matters related to health status. To participate effectively in decision making, patients must be encouraged to take responsibility for requesting additional information or clarification about their health status or treatment when they do not fully understand information and instructions. Patients are also responsible for ensuring that the health care institution has a copy of their written advance directive if they have one. Patients are responsible for informing their physicians and other caregivers if they anticipate problems in following prescribed treatment.

Patients should also be aware of the hospital's obligation to be reasonably efficient and equitable in providing care to other patients and the community. The hospital's rules and regulations are designed to help the hospital meet this obligation. Patients and their families are responsible for making reasonable accommodations to the needs of the hospital, other patients, medical staff, and hospital employees. Patients are responsible for providing necessary information for insurance claims and for working with the hospital to make payment arrangements, when necessary.

A person's health depends on much more than health care services. Patients are responsible for recognizing the impact of their life-style on their personal health.

CONCLUSION

Hospitals have many functions to perform, including the enhancement of health status, health promotion, and the prevention and treatment of injury and disease; the immediate and ongoing care and rehabilitation of patients; the education of health professionals, patients, and the community; and research. All these activities must be conducted with an overriding concern for the values and dignity of patients.

"A Patient's Financial Bill of Rights"

(What Medical Consumers Really Need)

The consumer protections contained in "A Patient's Financial Bill of Rights" should give the patient the power over hospitals and physicians in billing transactions.

1. **Patients must receive itemized bills for all charges.** Patients have a right to an itemized bill, in plain language, with a clear description of each item for which the patient is being charged.

2. **Patients must have access to medical records.** Patients or their assigned representatives shall receive one copy of medical records free of charge upon written request. Such a written request must be honored within 15 days. Patients must have the right to verify the accuracy of their bills.

3. **Providers must answer all patient inquiries regarding their bills.** Facilities must be available during normal business hours to receive inquiries

regarding charges. Written responses must be made within a reasonable time frame (5 business days).

4. Patients are not responsible for erroneous or un-documented charges. If a patient disputes a provider's charge, the provider must investigate the charge in question and make the proper adjustment to the patient's account within 30 days. If adjustments are not made, proper documentation supporting the charges should be supplied in writing within 30 days.

5. Patients cannot be required to make payments on disputed charges. Disputed items must be separately itemized on subsequent bills until the disputed charges are verified and resolved. Late charges cannot be added while charges are in dispute.

6. Providers cannot turn patient accounts over to a collection service if the patient is disputing or investigating charges. Facilities cannot report patients to a credit bureau as being deliquent if charges are in dispute.

7. Providers must pay interest and damages. If a patient has made payments toward any incorrect charges, the facility must refund the incorrect charges plus interest to the patient. In addition, any provider that assesses unlawful charges to patients will be subject to damages of $1,000.00

per violation, plus any expense incurred to resolve the overcharges.

8. Patients must be notified in writing of any credits they may have on their patient account. The
provider must notify the patient within 14 days
of any credits and offer the patient the choice of
either receiving a refund check or having the refund credited to the patient's remaining balance
or future charges.

9. Patients have the right to use outside agencies
to act on their behalf to help them resolve
charges with providers, with no additional re-
strictions or penalties.

10. Patients have the same rights above with regards
to insurance companies. Insurance companies
must supply written documentation to support
denials.

Appendix A

Online Resources
A Directory of Helpful Web Sites

While the following is by no means an exhaustive listing of medical and insurance related Web sites, I've found these sites useful to me personally. Many of these pages present different paths to the same information (more or less), and I suggest you find the ones that best meet your specific needs and purposes.

Rather than attempt to prioritize them or rate their worth, I've just alphabetized them within each category:

GENERAL MEDICAL INFORMATION AND SEARCH ENGINES

Site
　　Location

CliniWeb International
　　http://www.ohsu.edu/cliniweb/

drkoop.com
>http://drkoop.com

Health Information Resources Keyword Listing
>http://nhic-nt.health.org/AlphaKeyword.htm

HealthAtoZ: The Source for Health and Medicine
>http://www.healthatoz.com/

InteliHealth Professional Network
>http://ipn.intelihealth.com

Mayo Clinic Health Oasis Information
>http://www.mayohealth.org/

Medical Matrix
>http://www.medmatrix.org/index.asp

Medscape Surgery
>http://www.medscape.com/home/topics/surgery/
>surgery.html

MedWeb
>http://www.medweb.emory.edu/MedWeb/

Online Atlas of Surgery
>http://www.mic.ki.se/Diseases/e4.html

ThriveOnline
>http://thriveonline.com

Yahoo! Health
>http://dir.yahoo.com/health/index.html

MEDICAL DICTIONARIES

Site
>**Location**

American Medical Association
>http://www.ama-assn.org/

drkoop.com Search
    http://www.drkoop.com/search/
Medical Dictionary
    http://medical-dictionary.com/
Merriam-Webster Medical Dictionary
    http://www.medical-dictionary.com/
The National Women's Health Information Center
    http://www.4woman.org/nwhic/references/
    dictionary.htm
Medical Dictionary Surgical Glossary
    http://www.mtdesk.com/d.shtml

MEDICAL PRODUCTS AND PROCEDURES

Site
   Location

Medical Product Manufacturers/Suppliers
    http://www.medmarket.com/indexes/ixlc_b.html
MEDMarket Internet Medical Products Guide
    http://impg.medmarket.com/
Online Laparoscopic Technical Manual
    http://www.laparoscopy.net/lapmenu.htm

MEDICATIONS (BRAND NAME AND GENERIC)

Site
   Location

1999 Preferred Drug List
    http://www.uhc.com/pharmacy

CIGNA HealthCare Drug List
> http://www.cigna.com/healthcare/formulary.html

Drug InfoNet
> http://www.druginfonet.com/phrminfo.htm

drugstore.com
> http://www.drugstore.com/pharmacy/drugindex/
> default.asp

Mayo PharmaCenter
> http://www.mayohealth.org/usp/di/uspA-AM.htm

PharmInfoNet DrugDB
> http://pharminfo.com/drugdb/db_mnu.html

RxList.com, Inc.
> http://www.rxlist.com/cgi/rxlist.cgi

Search DRUGS
> http://www.medscape.com/misc/formdrugs.html

STATE-BY-STATE CHARGES FOR
MEDICAL RECORDS

Site
> **Location**

American Health Information Management Association
> http://www.ahima.org/publications/2a/pract.brief.
> 0199a.html

INSURANCE INFORMATION

Site
   Location

Health Care Financing Administration
   http://www.hcfa.gov/
The Health Insurance Association of America
   http://www.hiaa.org
insure.com
   http://www.insure.com/
National Association of Insurance Commissioners
   http://www.naic.org/

Appendix B

If You Need Help
A DIRECTORY OF MEDICAL BILLING ADVOCATES OF AMERICA

If you'd like someone else to review your medical bills and insurance coverage for you, or you just need advice, please feel free to give our office a call. We have affiliates across the country to serve your needs.

Here's how you can reach us:

Medical Billing Advocates of America
P.O. Box 1705
Salem, VA 24153
Contact: Candy Turner
Phone: (540) 387-5870
Fax: (540) 387-5043
E-mail: MBAofAM@aol.com

The Medical Billing Advocates of America members directory (listed here alphabetically by state) is constantly adding new members. Contact the national association for the member closest to you.

ALABAMA

Insurers Guardian Inc.
225 Broad Street, Suite 400
Gadsden, AL 35901
Contact: Janice Jackson or Max and Bonnie Stinson
Phone: (256) 547-4755
Fax: (256) 549-0091
E-mail: InsurersGuardian@netscape.net

ARIZONA

Alpha-Logic Inc.
2968 W. Ina Road, PMB 230
Tucson, AZ 85741
Contact: Mark Finchem
Phone: (520) 219-5118 or (800) 484-3955, ext. 4859
E-mail: alphalogic@juno.com
(Offices also in Holland, MI; Dallas, TX; Seattle, WA;
    and Indianapolis, IN)

CALIFORNIA

Accuracy in Medical Billing
500 San Nicholas Ct.
Laguna Beach, CA 92651
Contact: Renee Lucido
Phone: (949) 497-1005

Fax: same
Email: renee2chr714@aol.com

GEM Healthcare Business Consultants
1751 Beryl Street
San Diego, CA 92109
Contact: Goedela Robbins
Phone: (858) 274-4409
Fax: (208) 728-1916
E-mail: gemofsd@yahoo.com

MedBill Recovery Inc.
33585 Via De Agua
San Juan Capistrano, CA 92675
Contact: Jeffery L. Morgan
Phone: (949) 443-2024
Fax: (949) 443-9018
E-mail: j_morgan@ix.netcom.com

Sterling Enterprises
1756 Rosevilla
Pasadena, CA 91106
Contact: David Chick
Phone: (909) 971-2241
Fax: (413) 581-0957
E-mail: mchick@earthlink.net

WestMed Data Management
1660 W. Stuart Ave.
Fresno, CA 93711-1955
Contact: Sean Ford and Allen Lee
Phone: (559) 448-9752 (Sean) (559) 431-1509 (Allen)
E-mail: sfordrb@aol.com or rbdad1952@aol.com (Sean)
        leetwo@pacbell.net (Allen)

COLORADO

Eagle Eye Medical Recovery
743 Horizon Ct., Suite 342
Grand Junction, CO 81506
Contact: Art Lund
Phone: (970) 242-8243
Fax: (970) 242-8243
E-mail: alund@gj.net
Web site: http://shrinkmybills.com

MedAudit Services
2585 Heathrow Dr.
Colorado Springs, CO 80920
Contact: Linda Larkin
Phone: (719) 265-8767
Fax: (719) 264-9796
E-mail: MedAuditsv@aol.com

MedSave Services
P.O. Box 63084
Colorado Springs, CO 80962
Contact: Beverly Velte
Phone: (719) 592-1172
Fax: (978) 285-6556
E-mail: bbueno@msn.com
Web site: http://members.xoom.com/medsave/

Sand Creek Healthcare Auditing & Consulting
34153 Pinto Ct.
Elizabeth, CO 80107
Contact: Vivian Christensen
Phone: (303) 646-1731
(303) 265-9709 voice mail
Fax: (303) 265-9709
E-mail: vachris_1999@yahoo.com

DELAWARE

MDS (Medical Documentation Specialist)
610 Tolham Drive
Bear, DE 19701
Contact: Lois Sullivan
Phone: (302) 834-1474
Fax: (302) 834-4257
E-mail: Lsully21@hotmail.com

FLORIDA

Equity Medical Services
1613 Lahaina Court
Gulf Breeze, FL 32561
Contact: Sandra Klee
Phone: (850) 932-5290
Fax: (850) 916-1386
E-mail: sandra_klee@hotmail.com

MRCE (Medical Recovery and Consulting Experts)
P.O. Box 1163
Oldsmar, FL 34677-1163
Contact: Debra P. Lupe
Phone: (813) 818-8777
Fax: (813) 818-8777
E-mail: mrce@wans.net

GEORGIA

Medical Refund Service
P.O. Box 671987
Marietta, GA 30006

Contact: Cindy Holtzman
Phone: (770) 952-6284
Fax: (770) 955-0871
E-mail: mdrefund@bellsouth.net

ILLINOIS

Medical Bill Recovery
271 First Street
Granite City, IL 62040
Contact: Sarah McFadden
Phone: (618) 877-8326
Fax: (618) 877-9167
E-mail: mbrmcfadden@earthlink.net

Nichols & Jones Services
P.O. Box 25
Albion, IL 62806
Contact: Carolyn Nichols
Phone: (618) 445-9019
Fax: (618) 445-3642
E-mail: cnichols@wworld.com

IOWA

Medical Savings Specialists
P.O. Box 231
Winterset, Iowa 50273
Contact: Marcia Harris or Rebekah Mitchell
Phone: (515) 462-4337
Fax: (877) 694-0510
E-mail: rmitchell@gateway.net or marciaday@msn.com

KANSAS

R&D Associates
1330 Indian Rock Lane
Salina, KS 67401
Contact: Donna Swanson
Phone: (785) 825-6090
Fax: (785) 668-2605
E-mail: donlee@midusa.net or rvhalsey@midusa.net

KENTUCKY

Medical Consulting Services
621 South 2nd Street
Mayfield, KY 42066
Contact: Michelle Clay or Randy Adams
Phone: (270) 274-4444
Fax: (270) 274-4134
E-mail: mcs@mcsfirm.com
Web site: www.mcsfirm.com

Medical Review Services LLC
8502 Malibu Drive, Suite B
Louisville, KY 40219
Contact: Carol Cornett
Phone: (502) 968-8062
Fax: (502) 968-2872
E-mail: CCorn16466@aol.com

LOUISIANA

HealthMed Plus, Inc.
4217 Cleveland Place, Suite B

Metairie, LA 70003
Contact: Mary Reese
Phone: (504) 780-7222
Fax: (504) 780-7333
E-mail: RNFREE1006@aol.com

MARYLAND

Nightingales Medical Cost Management
1321 Riverside Pkwy E-2, PMB 126
Belcamp, MD 21017
Contact: Rosanne Dowdy
Phone: (410) 971-8213
E-mail: nightingales99@ivillage.com

MASSACHUSETTS

HCA (Healthcare Consumer Advocates)
56 Allston Street
Revere, MA 02151
Contact: David Bruno
Phone: (781) 284-8187
E-mail: dcbruno@email.msn.com

MICHIGAN

J. Kaufman & Associates LLC
30990 Westwood
Farmington Hills, MI 48331
Contact: Jack Kaufman
Phone: (248) 661-9800

Fax: (248) 661-9078
E-mail: JKAMEDICAL@aol.com

MISSOURI

Hefton & Associates, Inc.
14996 Nelly Dr.
Phillipsburg, MO 65722
Contact: Harold or Nancy Hefton
Phone: (417) 589-4315
Fax: (417) 589-4315
E-mail: nhefton@llion.org

NEW JERSEY

AW Benefits Consultants, Inc.
P.O. Box 16
Monmouth Junction, NJ 08852
Contact: Annette White
Phone: (732) 274-2563
Fax: (732) 438-8501
E-mail: awbenefits.com@worldnet.att.net

MedReview
879 West Park Ave. #176
Ocean, NJ 07712
Contact: Pamela Musico
Phone: (732) 869-1740
E-mail: snemerk@pol.net

NEW YORK

Metro Medical Claims Consulting Services
Empire State Building
350 Fifth Ave., Suite 3304 #7C
New York, NY 10118
Contact: Juan Valdivia
Phone: (973) 465-5390
Fax: (973) 465-8571
E-mail: jvaldivia@mindspring.com

NORTH CAROLINA

Betty Rowe & Associates
3267 Raleigh Street N.
Rocky Mount, NC 27801
Contact: Betty Rowe
Phone: (252) 977-9172
Fax: (252) 442-3941
E-mail: Roweaudit0@aol.com

Carolina Medical Solutions
P.O. Box 1084
Wrightsville Beach, NC 28480
Contact: Jill Bean
Phone: (910) 512-5976

Equitable Mediclaim Services
P.O. Box 1249
Pittsboro, NC 27312
Contact: Sue Bailes
Phone: (919) 545-2087
Fax: (919) 545-0257 (call first)
E-mail: mediclaim9@aol.com

OKLAHOMA

Health Audit Recovery Service
P.O. Box 2176
Elk City, OK 73648
Contact: Dora Martindale
Phone: (580) 225-6054
Fax: (580) 225-4848
E-mail: medaudit@hotmail.com

Medical Bill Review & Recovery
208 Russell Street
Hooker, OK 73945
Contact: Tim Hedrick
Phone: (316) 621-1906
Fax: (580) 652-3399

MEDPROBE Enterprises
P.O. Box 494
Mustang, OK 73064
Contact: Deb Pyland
Phone: (405) 376-5856
Fax: (405) 376-5857
E-mail: Medprobee@aol.com

PENNSYLVANIA

Edward R. Waxman & Associates
2677 Carnegie Road
York, PA 17402-3751
Contact: Edward Waxman
Phone: (717) 757-5613
Fax: (717) 997-7595
E-mail: erwaxman@usa.net

HealthCost Auditing LLC
2839 Benner Street
Philadelphia, PA 19149
Contact: Janet Bryant
Phone: (215) 743-9315
E-mail: janetbryant@earthlink.net

NEQIS Group
951 Richard Road
N. Huntingdon, PA 15642
Contact: Lisa Cohen
Phone: (412) 751-0552
Fax: (412) 751-5901
E-mail: neqis2@juno.com

Tracey Smeltzer
971 Midland Ave.
York, PA 17403
Phone: (717) 849-2141
Fax: (208) 275-0810
E-mail: traceysmeltzer@hotmail.com

RHODE ISLAND

Medical Recovery Service of New England LLC
PMB 227
580 Thames Street, Suite 227
Newport, RI 02840
Contact: Maridel Allen
Phone: (401) 847-4141
E-mail: MedicalRecovery.NewEngland@aya.yale.edu

SOUTH CAROLINA

Medical Billing Research Services
1035 Greenview Drive
Florence, SC 29501
Contact: Bob Hall
Phone: (843) 661-5356
Fax: (843) 661-6285
E-mail: hall.ruth@worldnet.att.net

SOUTH DAKOTA

Midwest Medical Auditing Inc.
Box 662, 802 S. River Street
Chamberlain, SD 57328
Contact: Terri Mohror
Phone: (605) 734-6249
E-mail: tmohror@easnet.net

TEXAS

Recovery Rx LLC
6723 Waggoner Drive
Dallas, TX 75230
Contact: Susan Spain
Phone: (214) 368-7998
Fax: (214) 368-7999
E-mail: recoveryrx@aol.com

VIRGINIA

Clark Group
5409 Studeley Ave.
Norfolk, VA 23508
Contact: Don Clark
Phone: (757) 489-4161
Fax: (757) 489-4161
E-mail: clarkgroup@hotmail.com

Medical Recovery Services Inc.
639 Catawba Dr.
Salem, VA 24153
Contact: Pat Palmer
Phone: (540) 387-2119
Fax: (540) 387-5043
E-mail: Medrecov@aol.com

Ron Hayes & Associates
13002 Walton Bluff Ct.
Midlothian, VA 23113
Contact: Ron Hayes
Phone: (804) 897-5280
Fax: (804) 378-5224
E-mail: RHayes1994@aol.com

WASHINGTON

Nationwide Medical Auditors
2918 NW Lower River Rd.
Vancouver, WA 98660
Contact: Barbara Coleman or Cindy Jaynes

Phone: (360) 735-0394
Fax: (413) 480-8743
E-mail: cjnationwide@aol.com and
   bcnationwide@juno.com

Bibliography

Androshick, Julie. "Hospital Robbery." *Forbes,* 22 April 1996, p. 219.

Better Business Bureau, Inc. *Better Business Bureau Literature—Health Insurance.* 1996. Internet. Available: www.bosbbb.org.

Davis, Neil M. *Medical Abbreviations: 8600 Conveniences at the Expense of Communications and Safety.* 9th ed. Neil M. Davis Associates, Jan. 1999.

Dolan, Ken, and Daria Dolan. "With Billing Errors Rampant, You Need Our Tips on How Not to Overpay for Medical Care." *Money,* Oct. 1995, p. 41.

Elsbach, Kimberly, Robert Sutton, and Kristine Principe. "Averting Expected Challenges through Anticipatory Impression Management: A Study of Hospital Billing." *Organizational Behavior* 9.1 (1998), pp. 68–86.

Foundation for Taxpayer & Consumer Rights. *The Bills Project.* 1999. Internet. Available: www.consumer-watchdog.org/public_hts/bills/.

Health Insurance Association of America. *HIAA Guide to*

Health Insurance. 1999. Internet. Available: www.hiaa. org.

Insurance News Network LLC. *insure.com: The Consumer Insurance Guide*. 1995–1996. Internet. Available: www.insure.com.

Jensen, Mike. "Red Tape." *NBC Nightly News*. NBC, New York, 29 May 1995.

Koop, C. Everett. "Dr. Koop's Guide to Managed Care." *Reader's Digest*, September 1999, pp. 78–83.

Mark, Erika Reider, ed. "The Better Way: How to Find Mistakes in Your Medical Bills." *Good Housekeeping*, Jan. 1992, pp.159–60.

National Association of Insurance Commissioners. *National Association of Insurance Commissioners*. 1996–1999. Internet. Available: www.naic.org.

Neighmond, Patricia. "Healthcare Fraud II." *National Public Radio's Morning Edition*. NPR, Washington D.C., 28 May 1997.

Wallace, Chris. "Bill Buster: Woman Helps Others Reduce Their Hospital Bills" *PrimeTime Live*. ABC News, New York, 4 Feb. 1998.

Index

Page numbers of illustrations appear in italics.